101

Things to Think

About

While Walking

Dan Walker

More from the Author

The Walking Plan: 30 Walking Challenges to Help

You Get Fit and Stay Healthy for Life

https://www.amazon.com/dp/B0C9HL76MJ

Introduction

Walking is a great way to stay in shape and improve your mental and physical well-being. Ever since the dawn of time, early humans have walked the Earth and populated the entire planet without relying on any form of modern-day transportation: no automobiles, no airplanes, no trains, and no ships. It's remarkable what a pair of feet can do!

Benefits of Walking

If there is one thing you can do every day from here on out to stay fit, it's to walk a few steps every day. Even if you can't walk a mile without taking a rest, it's better to walk a little bit at a time, say 15 minutes, than sit behind your desk or on the couch all day long. Over time, those little walks will add up, and soon you'll find yourself walking longer and longer. Within a year, you will see a gradual transformation in your health, body, diet, sleep, and mental attitude. There will come a day when you will feel confident enough to pursue big life goals you once thought were way out of reach. All it takes is putting one foot in front of the other.

Now, let's get walking!

How to Use This Little Book

Here are 101 intriguing questions to consider while walking. Believe it or not, intense thinking can burn calories! Roughly 10 to 15 calories are burned just by thinking intensely for 30 minutes. If you combine that with physical activity, such as walking, it can be as high as 20 to 25 calories. The more intelligent you are and the more complex your thoughts are, the more calories you will burn.

Granted, you can't think yourself into shape. But if you think intensely on a daily basis and over long stretches, those calories can add up over time, especially year after year.

Before each walk, pick a question (or two), either in the order presented or randomly. Once you have selected a question, spend 5 minutes thinking about what is being asked. These are not yes-or-no questions. Once you have pondered over the question long enough, answer it with a "because." Your response should take 10 minutes if you were to recite it to an audience. Each question takes about 15 minutes to complete. Pick as many as you like when you go for your daily walks.

Here's an example of how I would approach a question. You may have a different perspective. There is no right or wrong way; as long as you are putting in the mental effort is all that matters.

Do you consider yourself a good person, and do you have proof?

What do you mean by "good"? I noticed it says "yourself" and not others, so this is about self-reflection and not about what others think of me. Do I have to be good all the time, or can I just be good for 20 hours a day and slack off for 4 hours? Does that still make me a good person? Does being not-bad count towards being a good person? Like, I mind my own business and I don't pollute the air by smoking or coughing in public when I'm sick.

How good must I be to be at the optimal level of goodness? If I go overboard and become too good, then I have passed the point of diminishing returns. There is opportunity cost involved. So, in a way, I am harming myself by being overly good, and self-harm makes me a bad person.

I believe I am a good-enough person because I have lived my life, so far, as an upright and law-abiding citizen: I pay my taxes (state and federal), recycle and repair stuff, leave generous tips, and return borrowed things such as library books and shopping carts. If I were to die tomorrow, I could confidently say that my conscious is clear of any wrongdoing.

Some other reasons I believe I'm a good person: I like to think about ways to save the most number of lives with the least amount of effort; help others knowing they can't repay me; create an anonymous trust fund to benefit my local community; donate things I know families can't afford; and laugh at stupid jokes because someone needed to see a smile.

Well, you get the idea.

If you go on your walks with a friend, take a few

more questions along with you and decide which ones

to share. That way, you can see how well you truly

know each other.

101 Things to Think About While Walking

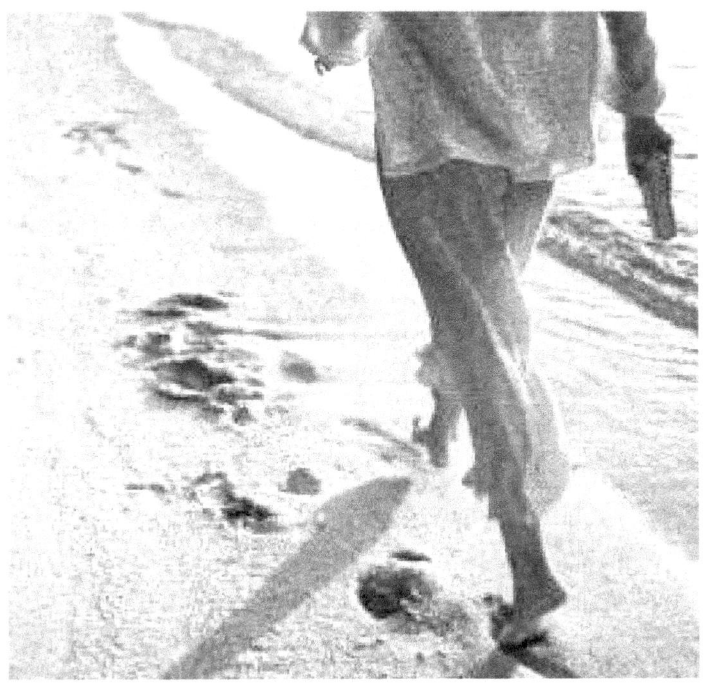

1. Is your existence an overall net positive or negative on the planet?

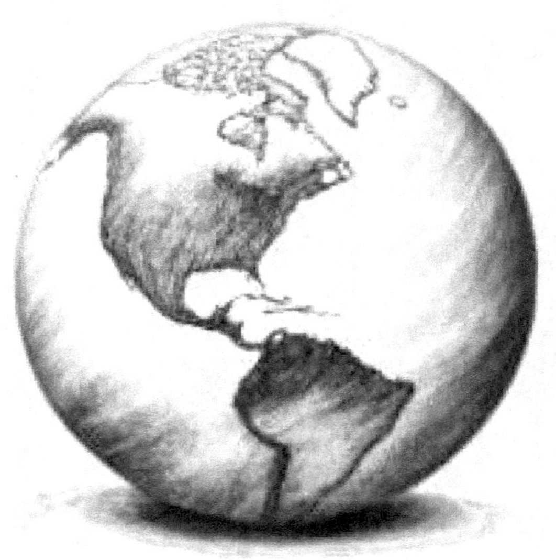

2. Do you consider yourself a good person, and do

you have proof?

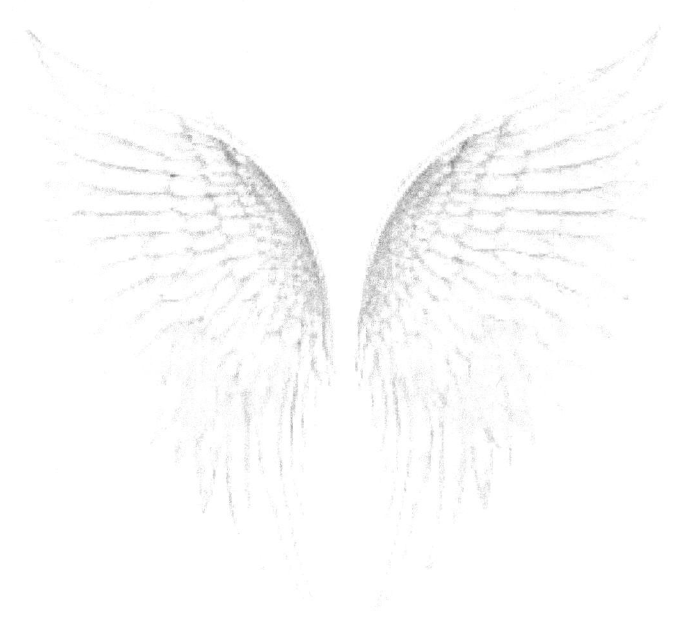

3. Have you ever said sorry first?

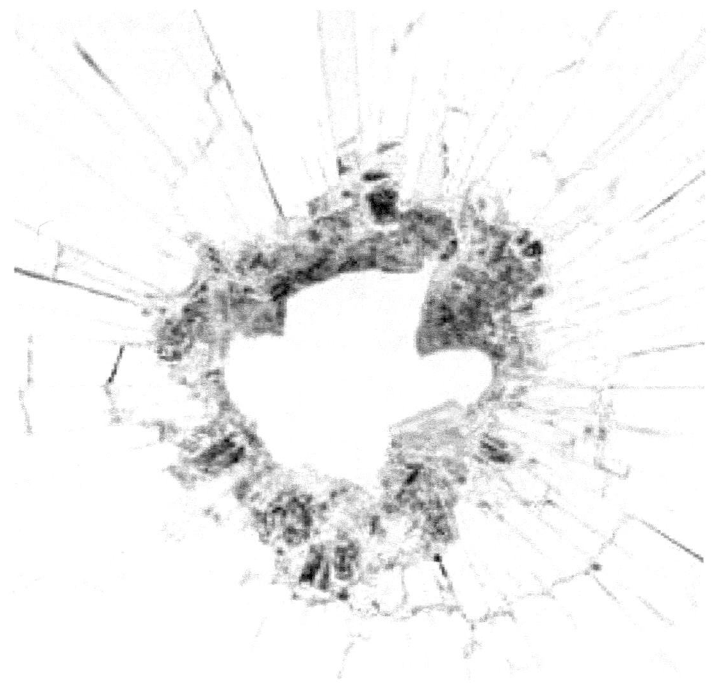

4. How much money do you think you need to never worry about money?

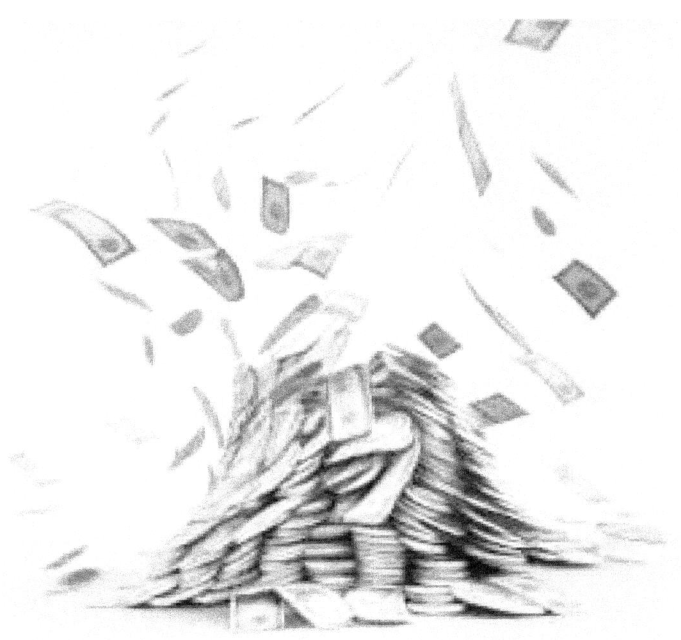

5. You are in a foreign country and don't speak the language and just met your soulmate. How would you communicate with this stranger?

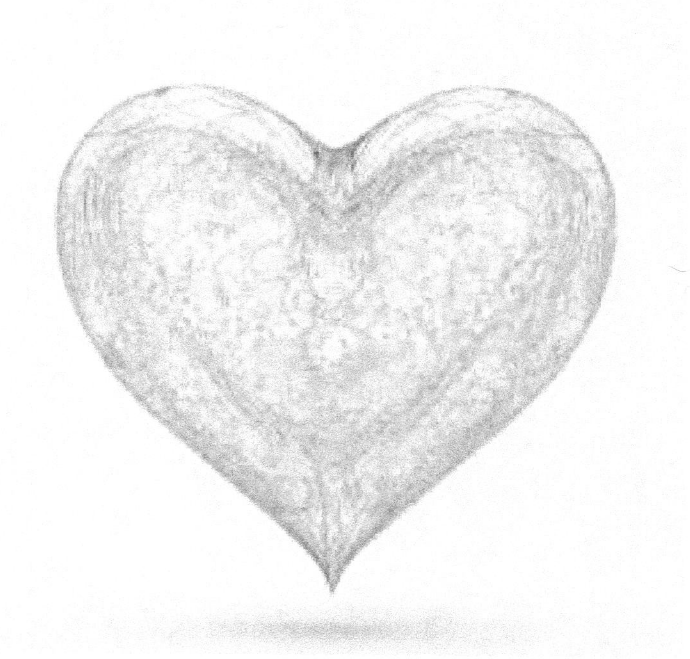

6. Name six people you met last week that brought a

smile to your face.

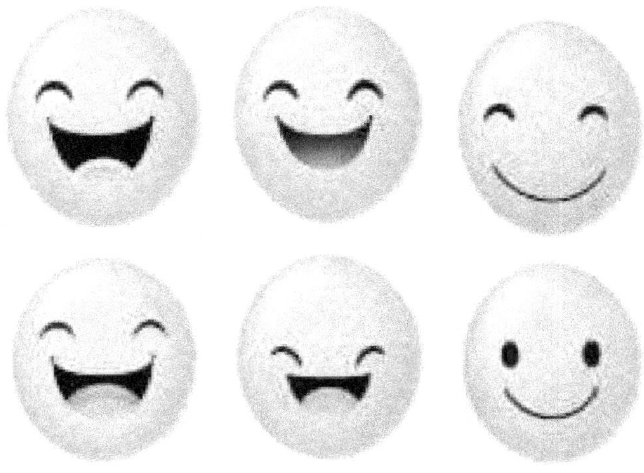

7. If you believe in the After Life, do you think you will

be allowed to pleasure yourself?

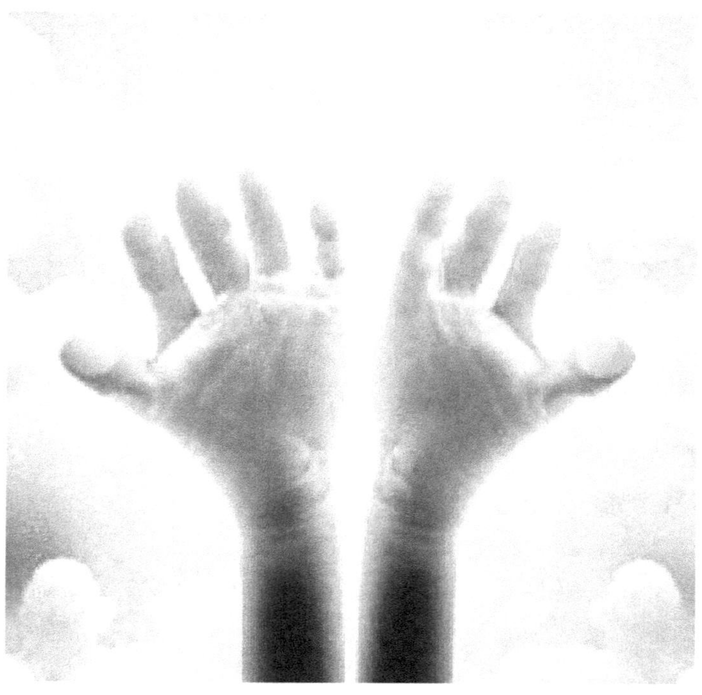

8. Which neighbor of yours do you think is a likely

suspect if the FBI came searching for a serial killer in

your neighborhood?

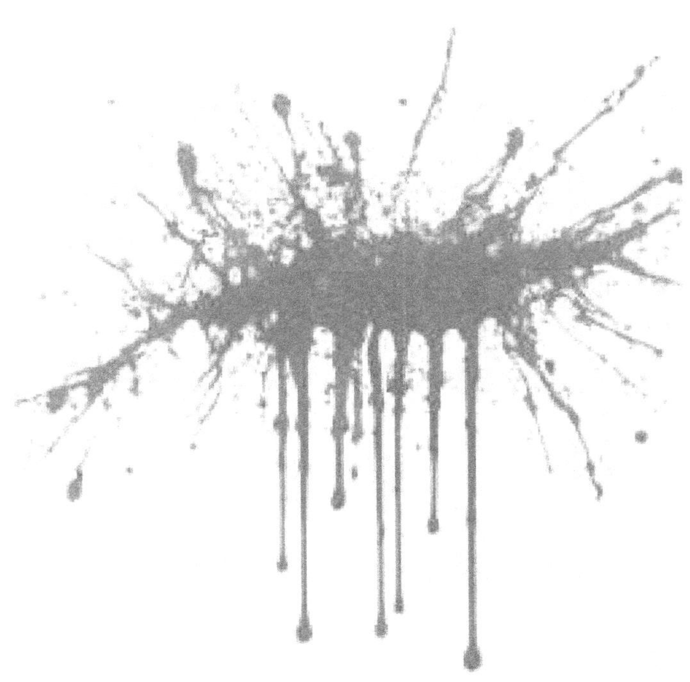

9. Do you believe there are truths in the universe beyond human understanding due to the physical size and constraints of the human brain?

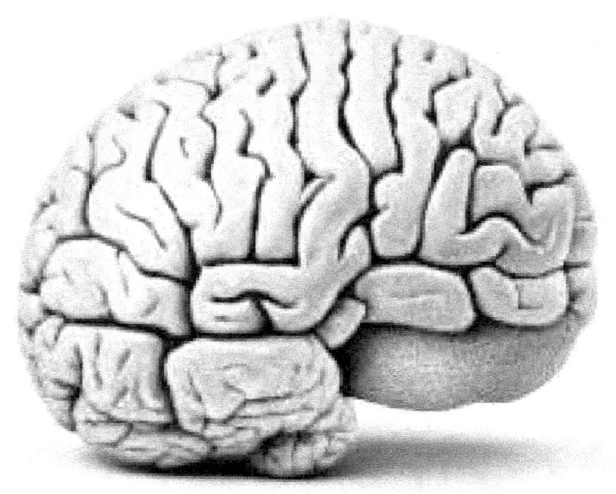

10. What is the one invention you cannot live without,

and would you trade your mother for it?

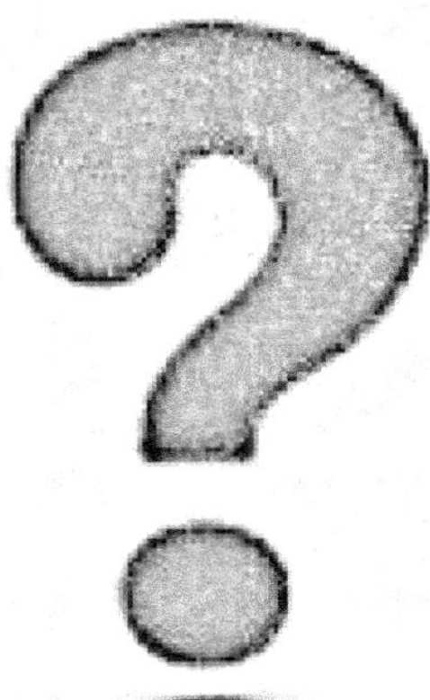

11. If you lost everything you own today, do you think

you can earn enough to get it all back?

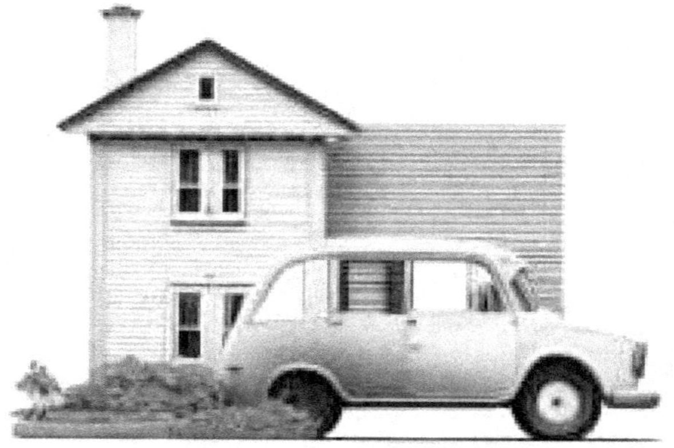

12. If you were of the opposite gender, would you see the world differently?

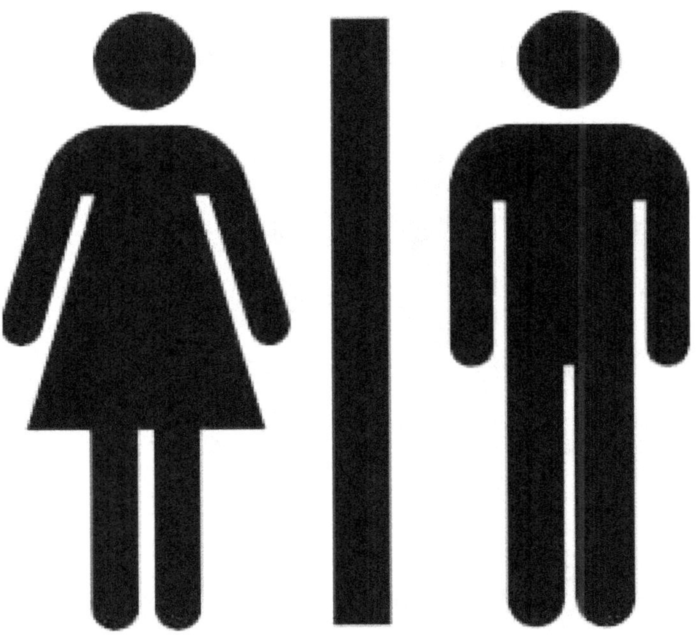

13. If you were a different ethnicity, would that change who you are?

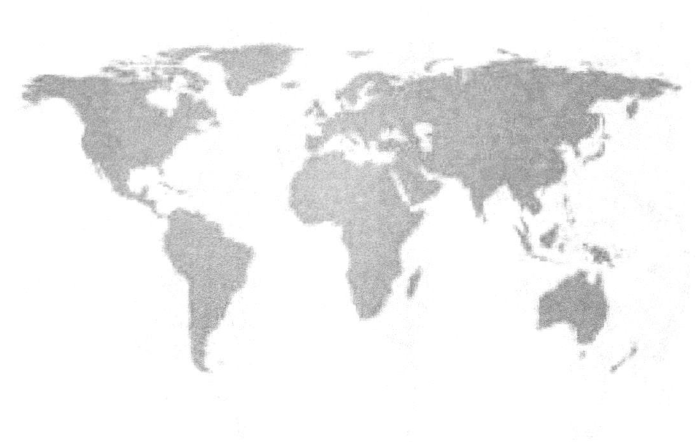

14. If you were stranded on an island, would you rather be with a beautiful person with an annoying voice or an ugly person with a beautiful voice?

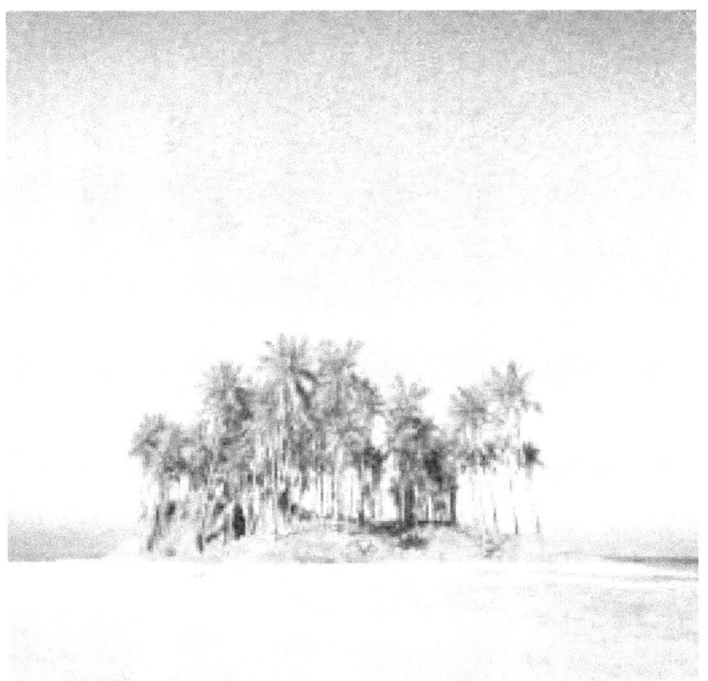

15. Would you rather spend a day in the city or a day
in the countryside with your mother-in-law?

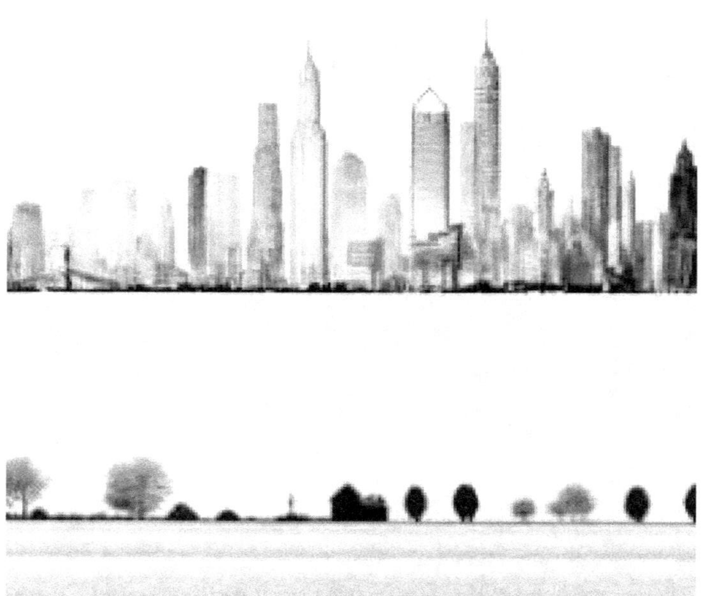

16. How many items of clothing do you think a normal person should own?

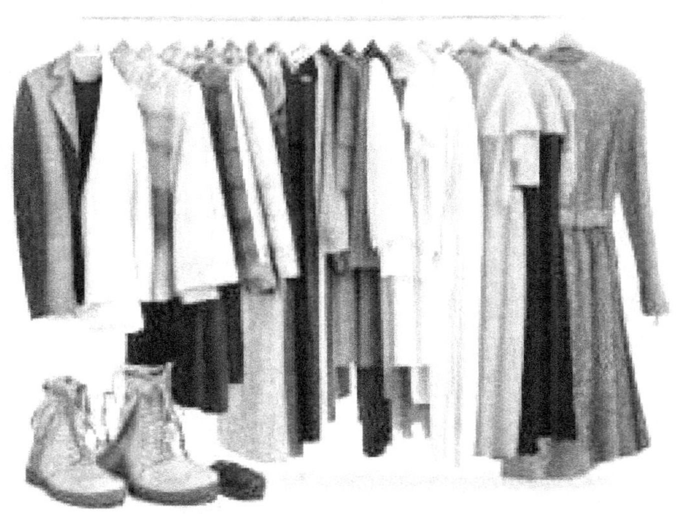

17. Name one physical aspect of your appearance that you don't like, and has anyone ever mention this to you?

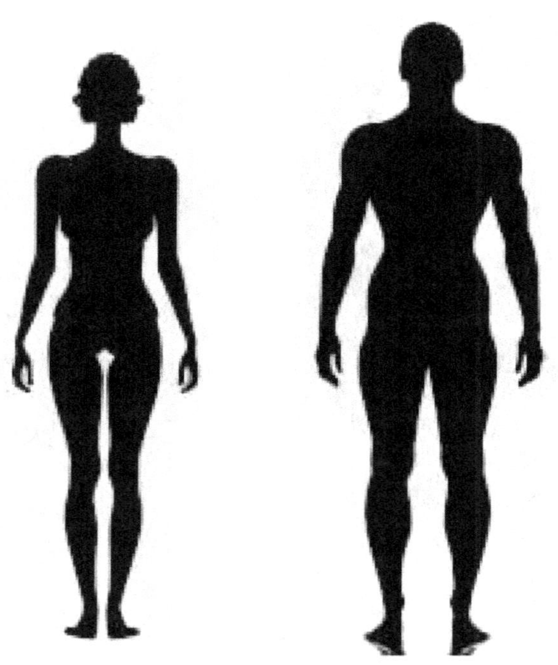

18. If you were to gain an extra 50 pounds, would you
consider yourself still attractive?

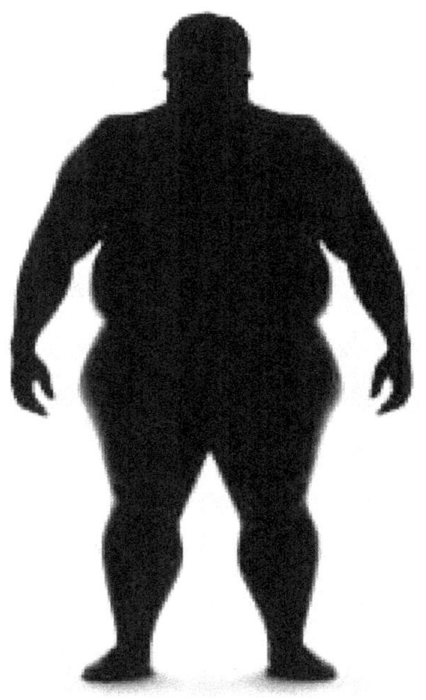

19. Do you think you have sufficient education and knowledge to make informed choices in the decades to come?

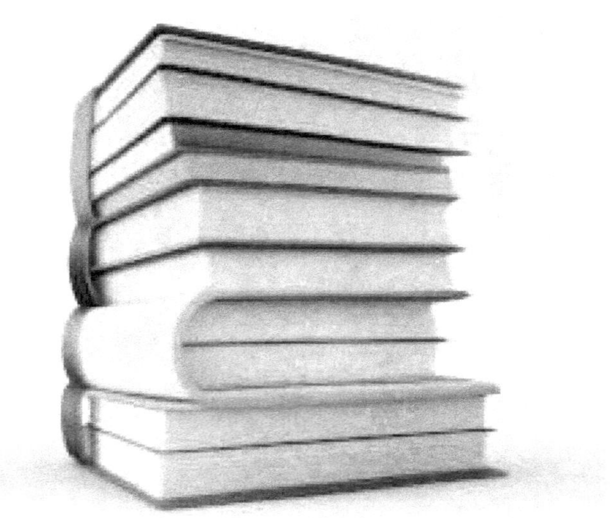

20. What one life skill do you think you still lack?

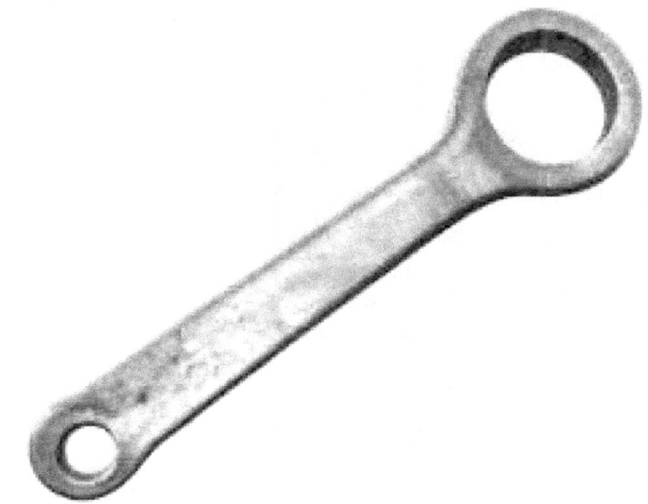

21. What is the biggest expense you wish you can cut
back but knows it will hurt your partner's feelings?

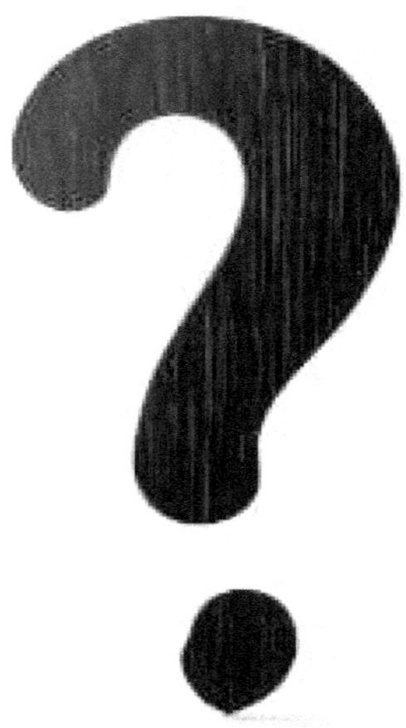

22. What do you plan to do for fun in your retirement?

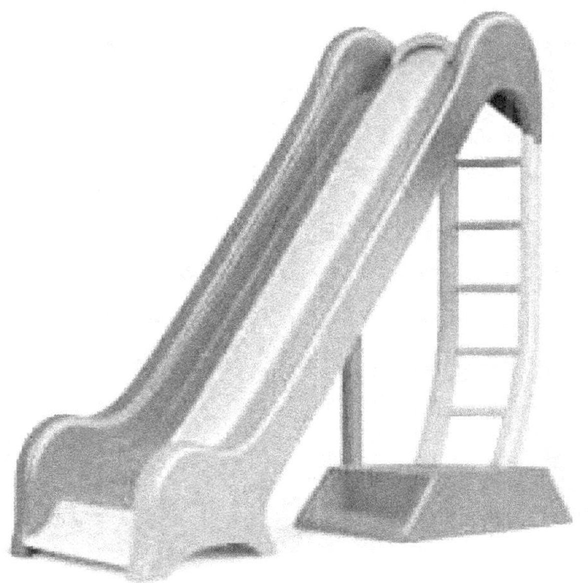

23. If you were to quit your job or school right now,

what would you be doing instead?

24. Would you rather have ten children or none at all,

if those were the only two options?

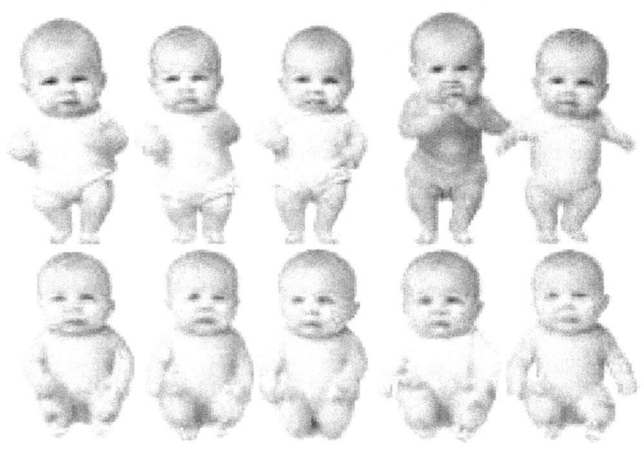

25. If you have just a year to live, who will you tell first?

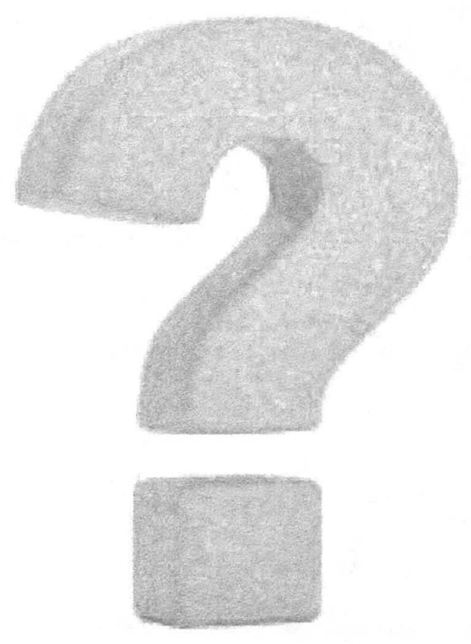

26. If you were to become permanently blind or deaf,

which one would you prefer?

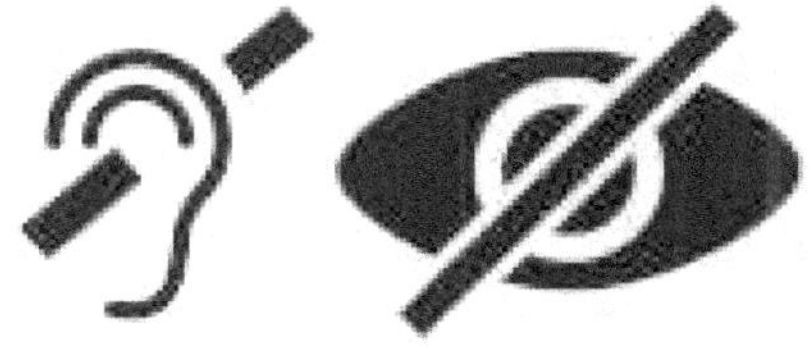

27. Which part of the day do you look forward to?

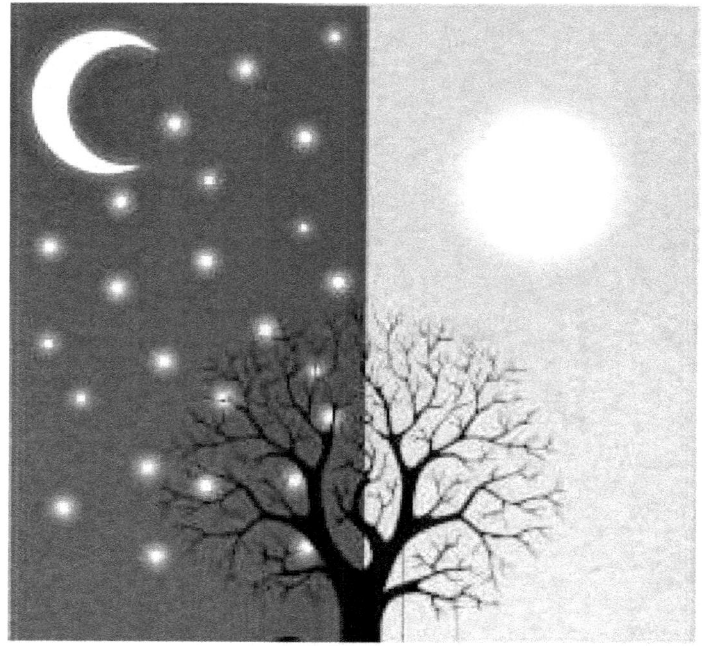

28. What activity do you think takes the most effort

and has the least payoff in terms of satisfaction?

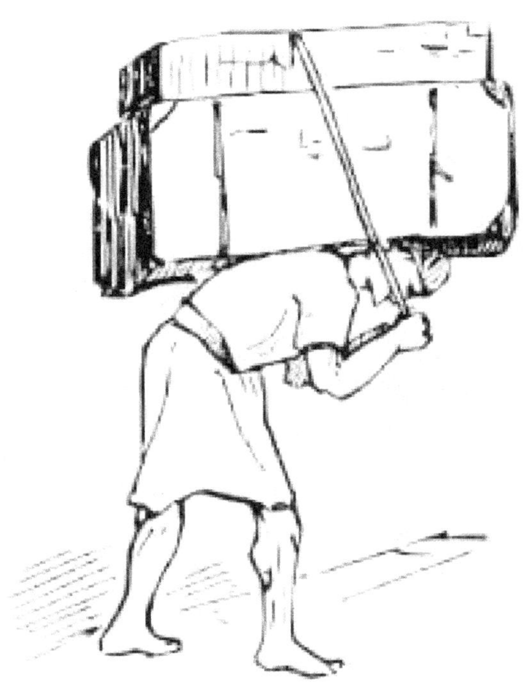

29. If you can only do one thing with your partner, would you rather do all the talking or listening?

30. Have you ever made a major life decision on an impulse?

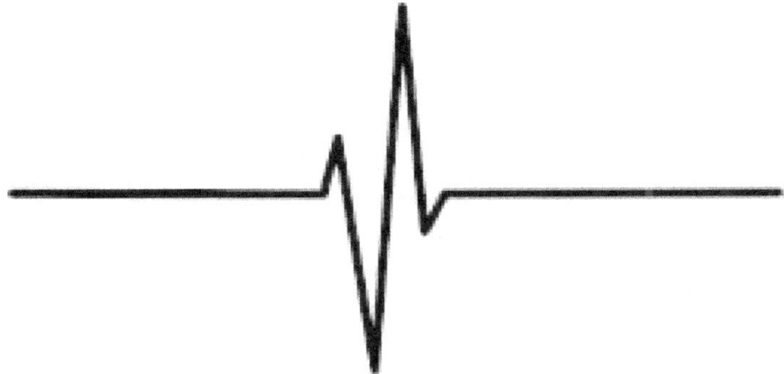

31. How far ahead or behind do you think you are in

the game of life?

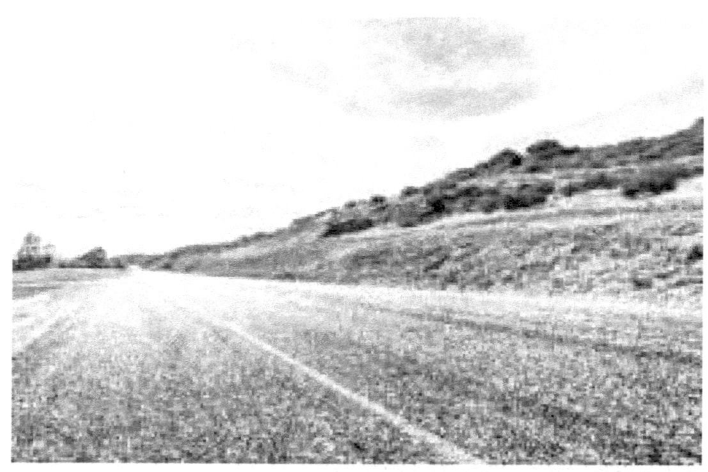

32. Can you recall any of your dreams you had last

week?

33. Would you rather have a friend who loves to make

you laugh or likes to listen to you talk all the time?

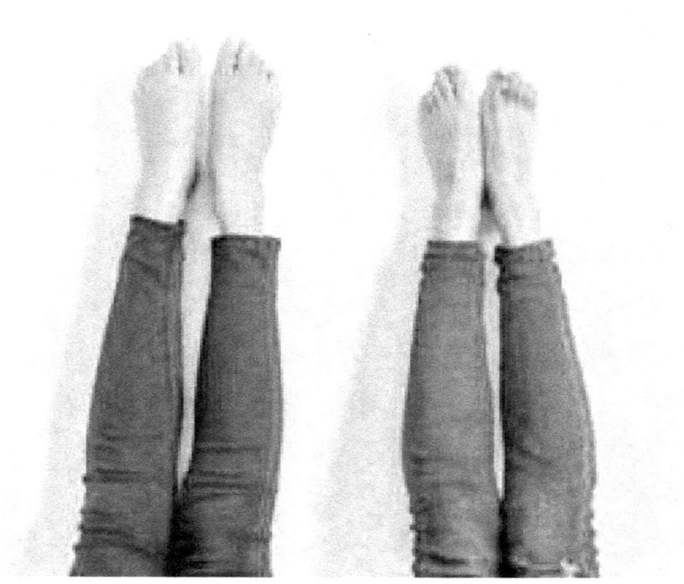

34. What is the one sport you wish you can play
professionally?

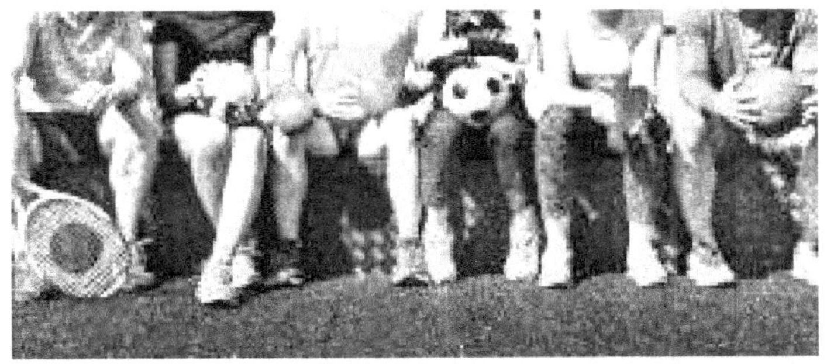

35. If you knew how much dedication and effort it took

to get where you are today, would you do it all over

again?

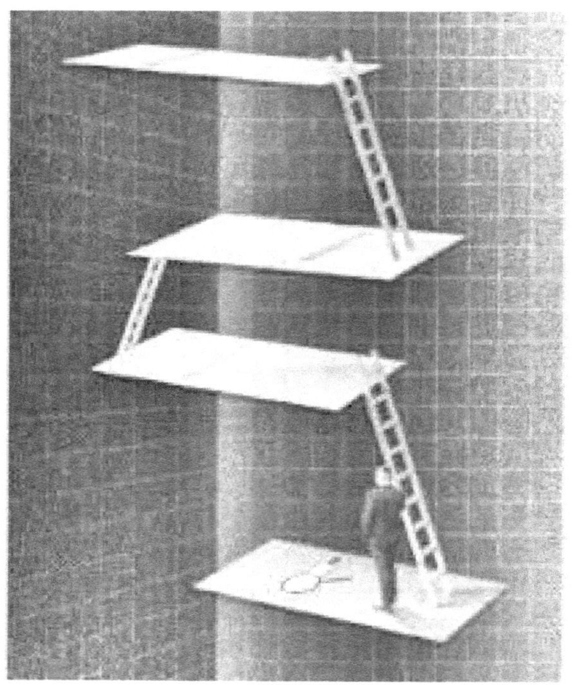

36. If you can play one musical instrument professionally in your career, which one will it be?

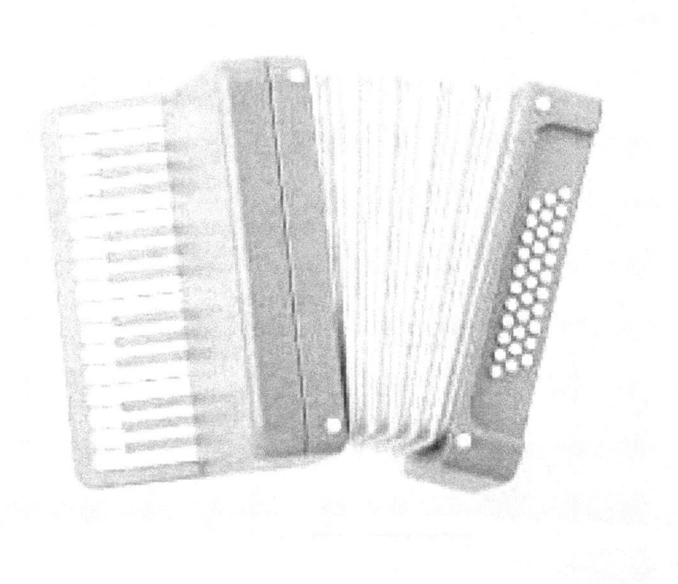

37. What smells bother you the most?

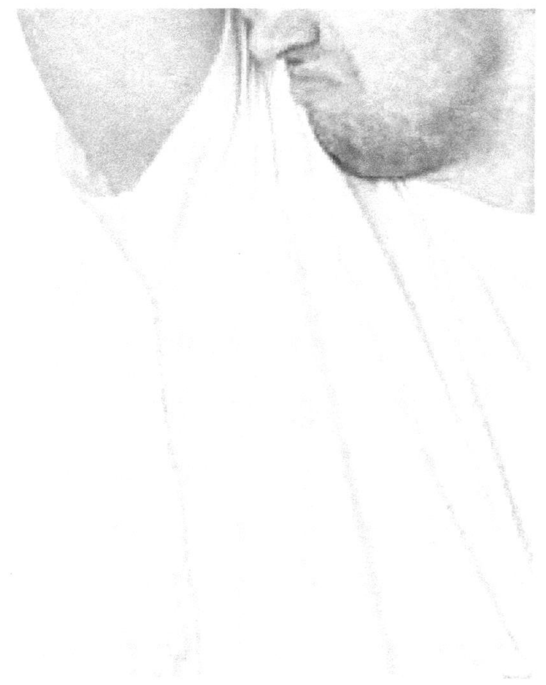

38. Are you aware of your own blind spots?

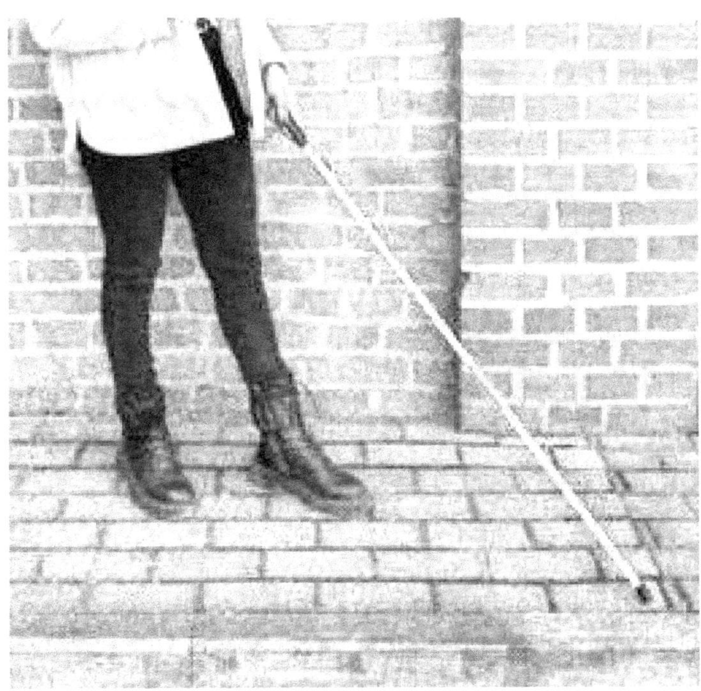

39. If you were to die tomorrow, who do you think will

be glad to see you go?

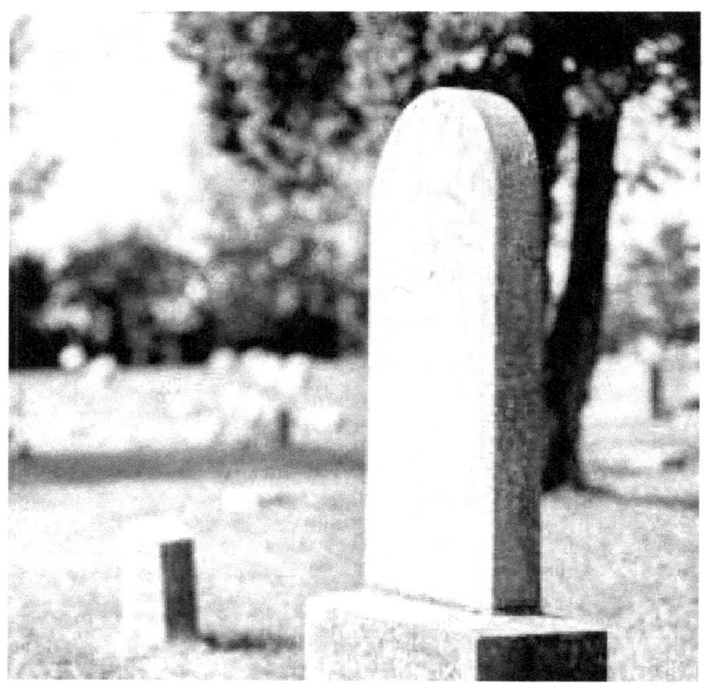

40. What are some beliefs you have that others
disapprove of?

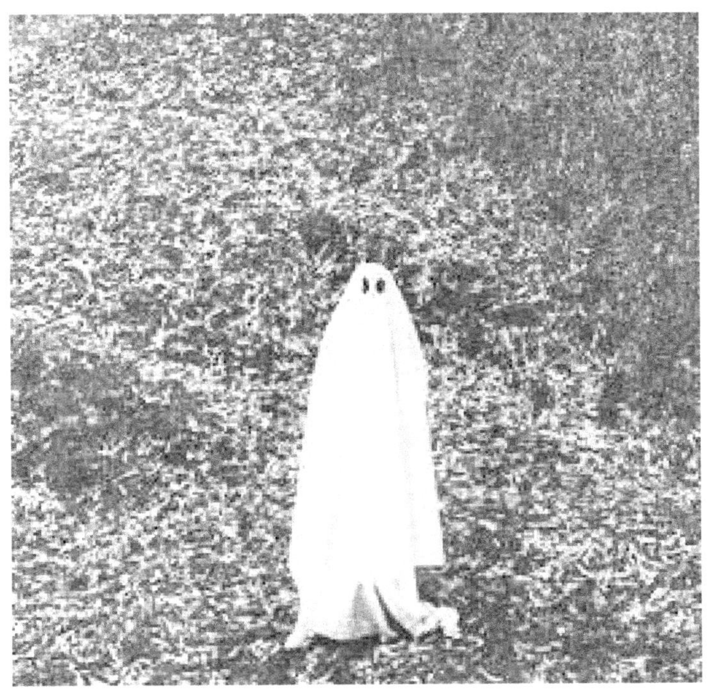

41. Can you remember what you wore to the last social event?

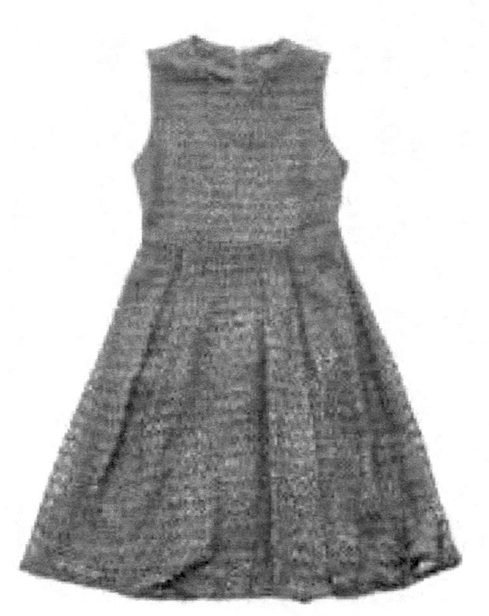

42. What would it take to motivate you to run for public office?

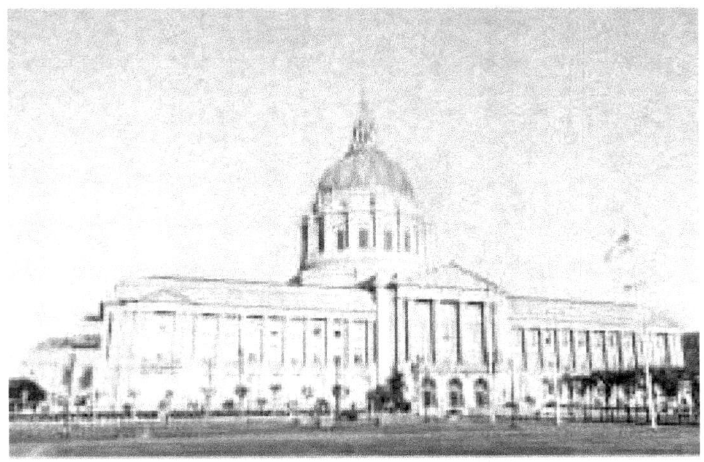

43. If you had a billion dollars, how would you spend it

all in your lifetime?

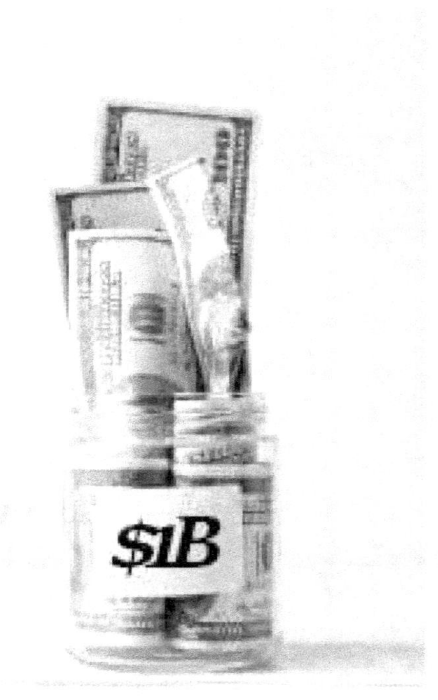

44. Recall the last time you were upset. When exactly

did you stop being upset?

45. How many lies do you hear on a daily basis?

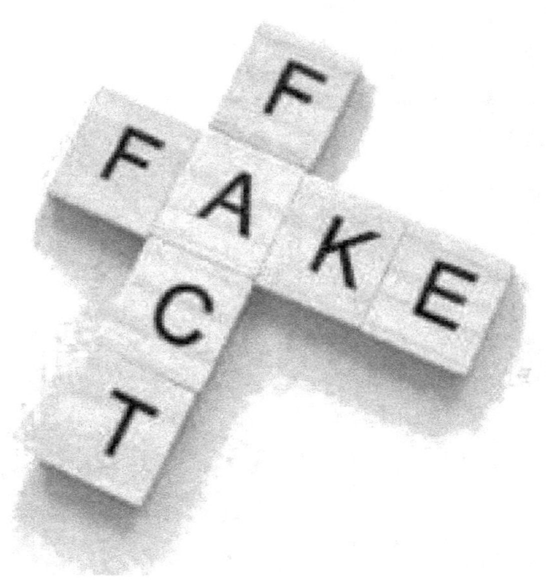

46. What one book would you like to memorize?

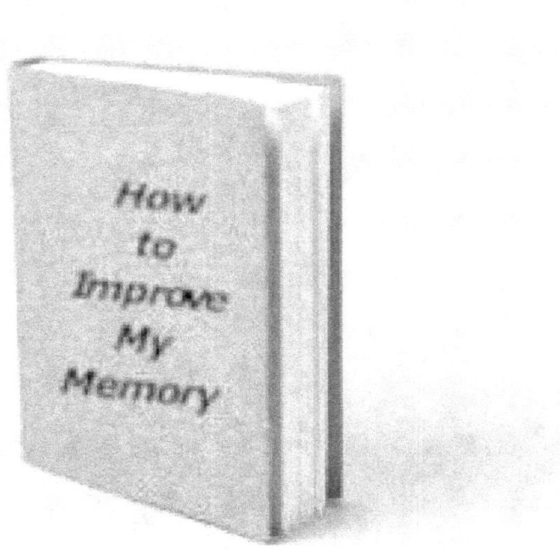

47. If you can donate your brain and live in someone else's body, would you do it?

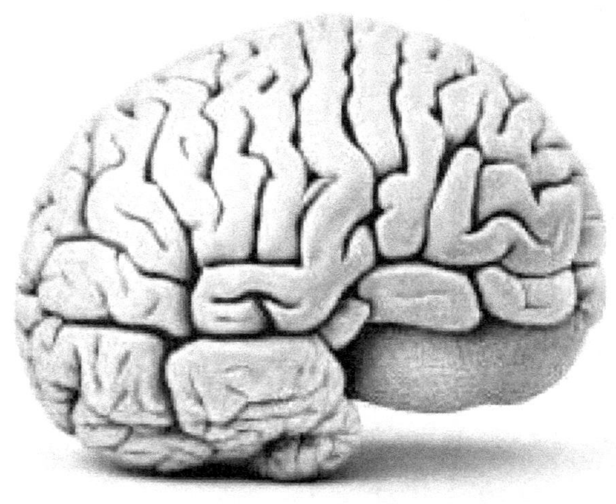

48. What is the most painful experience you ever have

to gone through?

49. Have you ever broken any hearts?

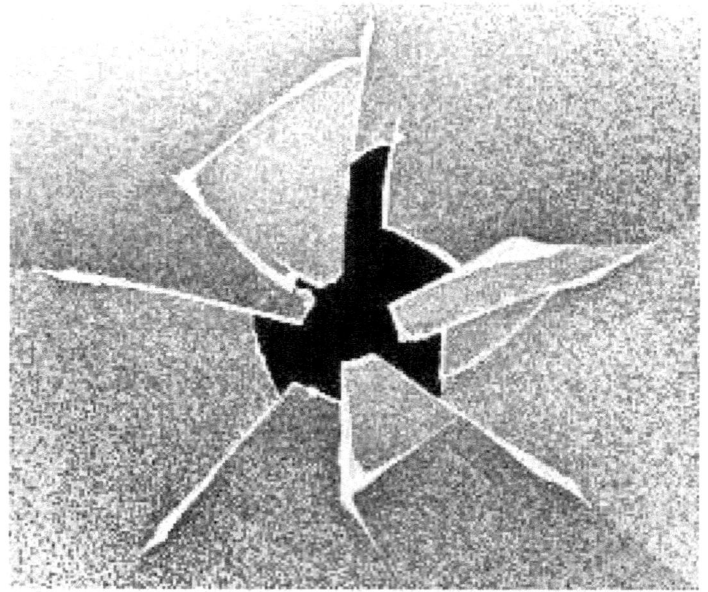

50. Is there anything you love so much that you would

sacrifice everything you have?

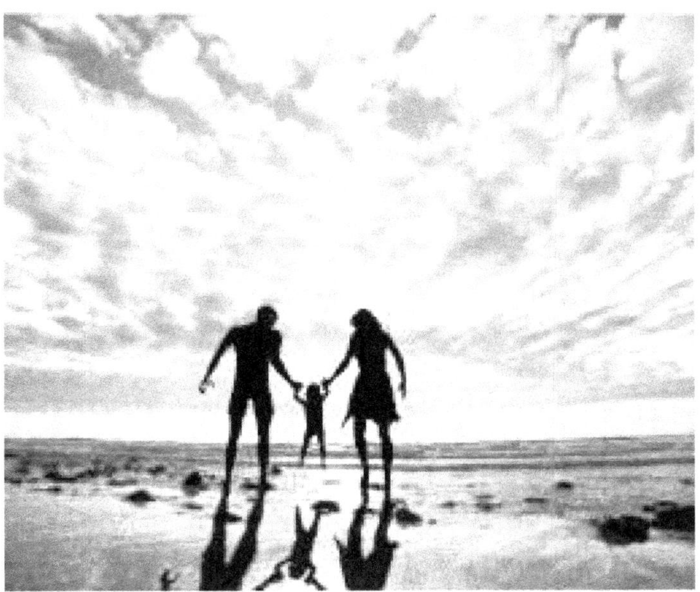

51. If you can do just one thing every day to make you

happy, what would it be?

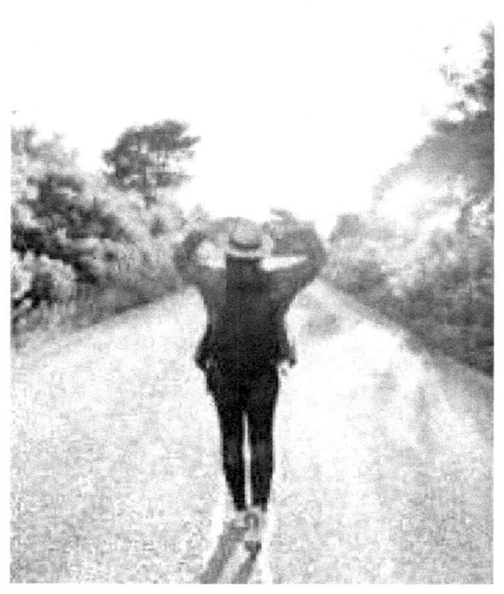

52. Do you think you are persistent enough in life?

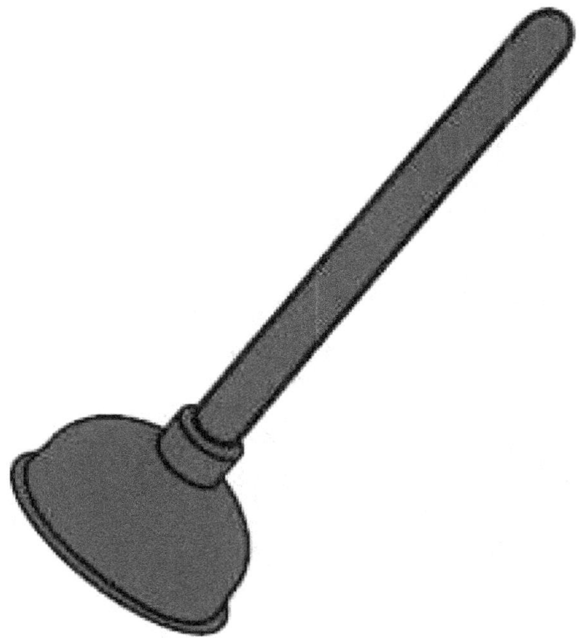

53. If you met a clone of yourself, would you have a
physical relationship with your clone?

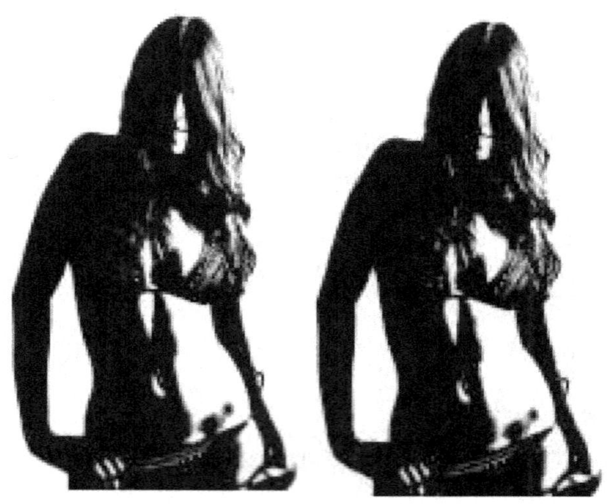

54. Do you owe your overall success in life to your

talent and hard work, or is it mostly due to luck?

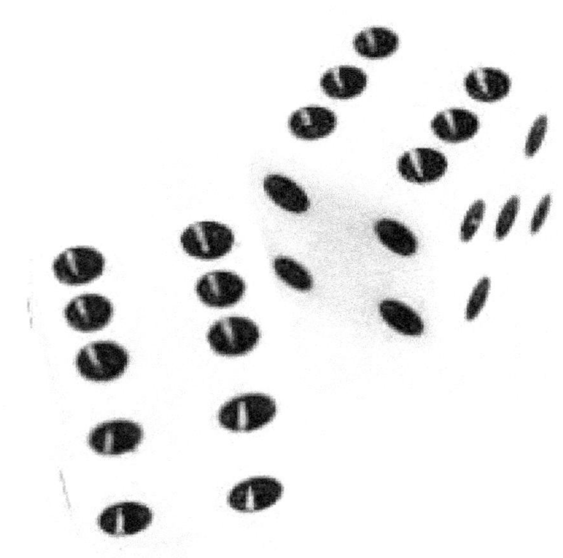

55. What do others admire the most about you, and

has anyone ever told you so?

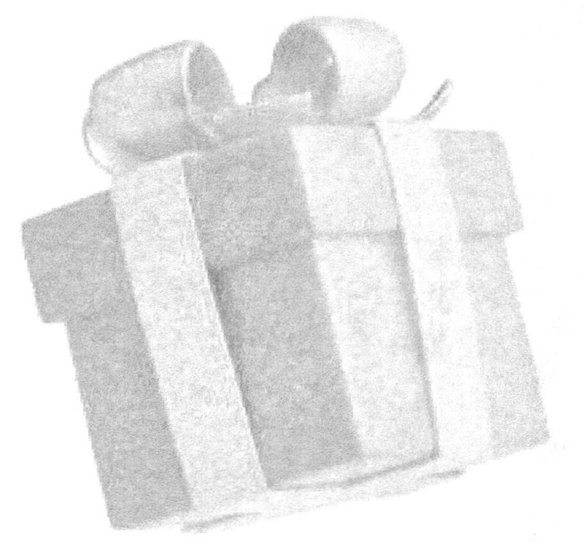

56. If you were to live to 100 years old, what accomplishments would you be most proud of?

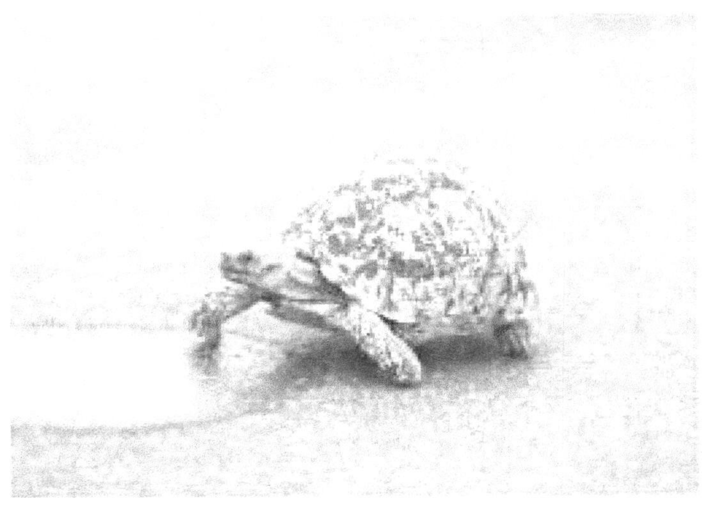

57. Think of the person you saw this week that you found repulsive. Now imagine being that person. How would you deal with people staring at you?

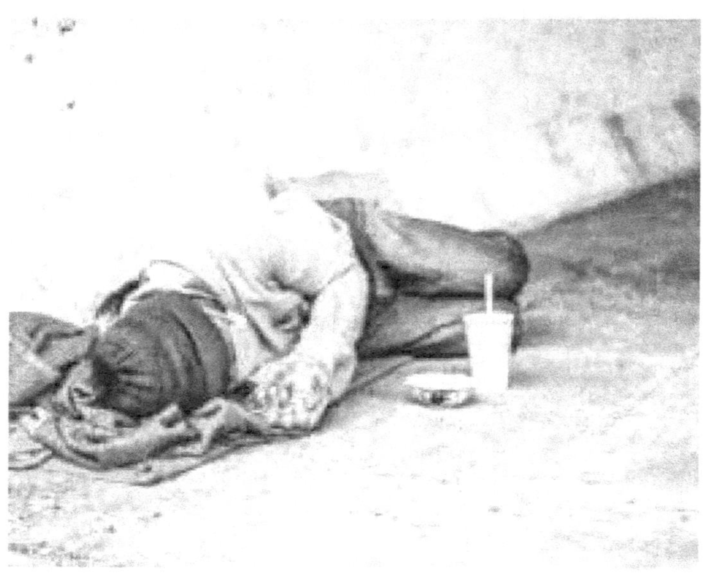

58. Think of the greatest year you ever had. Highlight

an event in every month of that year.

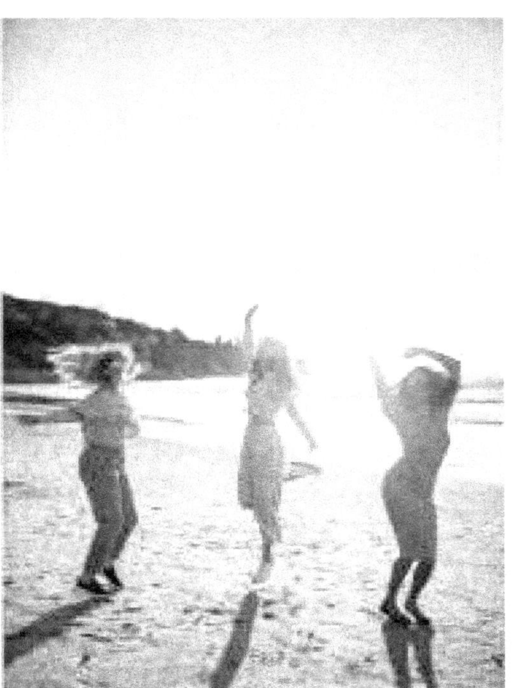

59. If you can relive 5 consecutive years of your life,

what years will you choose?

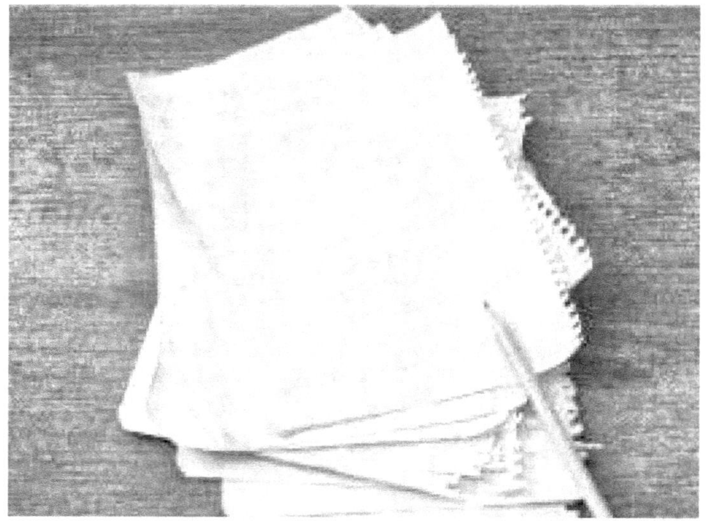

60. Think of a platonic friend that can be your life

partner. How would you win your friend over?

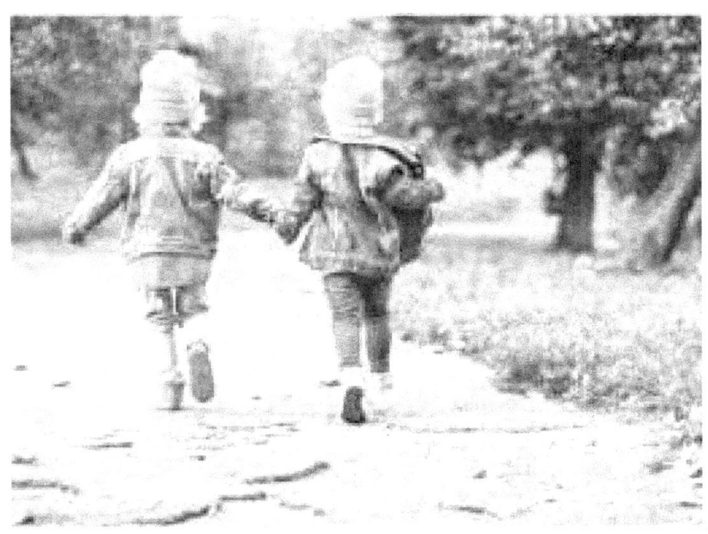

61. If movies were real, which movie would you want

to be in for the remaining years of your life?

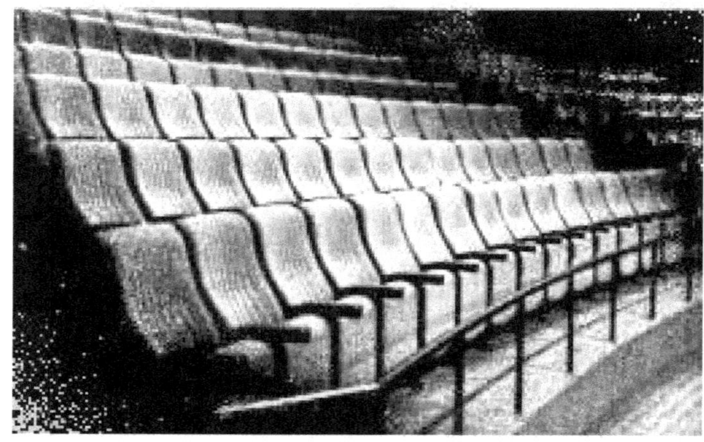

62. You are lost in the desert and had not eaten in days. Your pet just died a minute ago and you will soon follow. Would you rather die or eat your pet and be rescued?

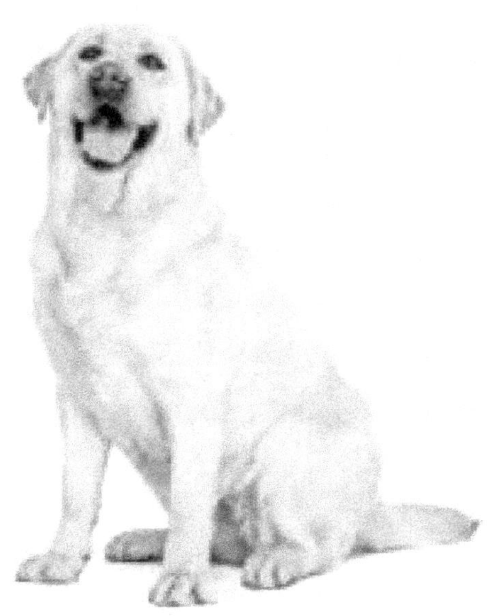

63. Is there one book you read that ultimately changed you to become who you are today?

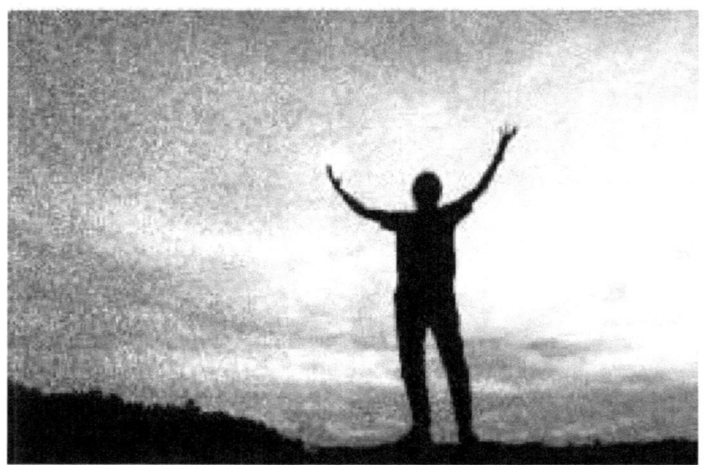

64. How many descendants do you think you'll have

500 years from now?

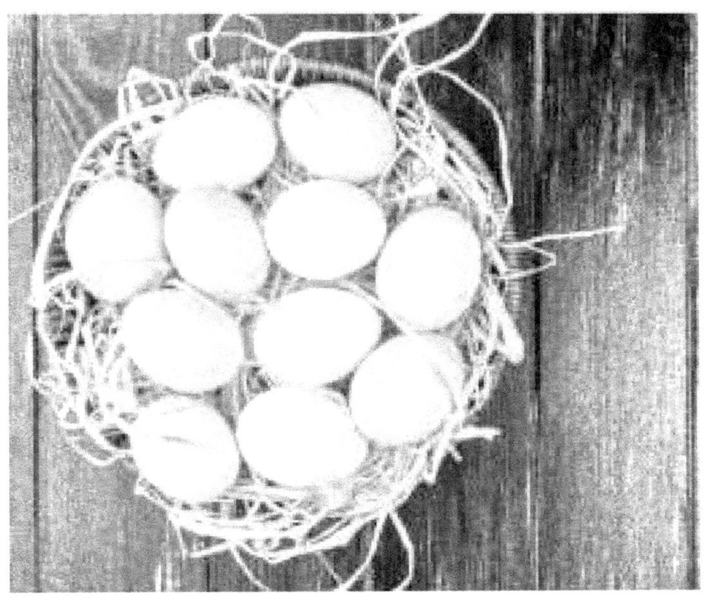

65. Do you know any of your neighbors' dreams?

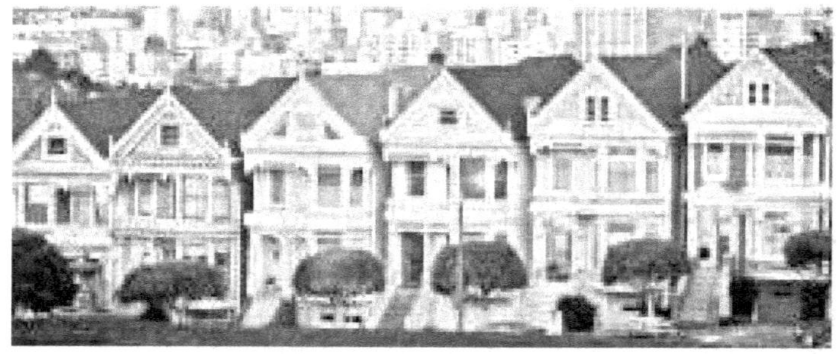

66. Do you want to know the exact date your partner
will pass away?

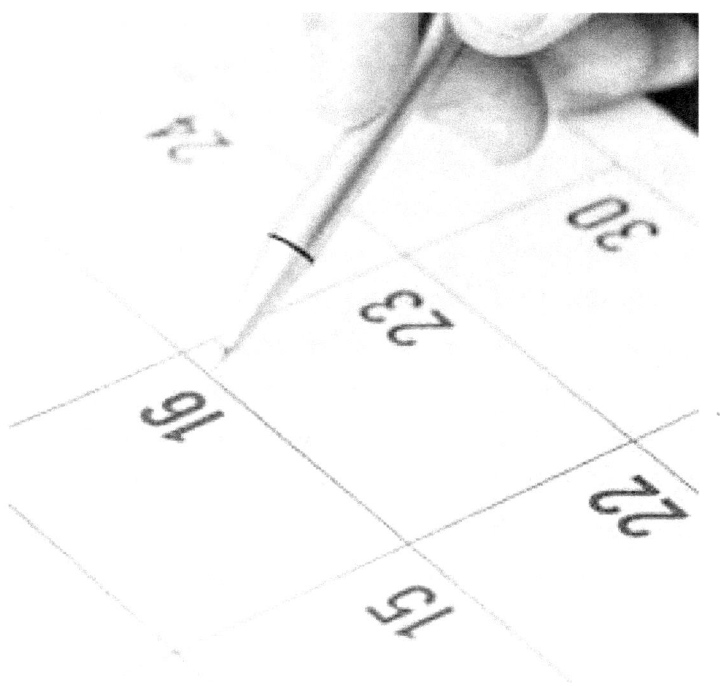

67. What one thing you do that annoys the hell out of
your partner?

68. What one thing your partner does that annoys you
the hell out of you?

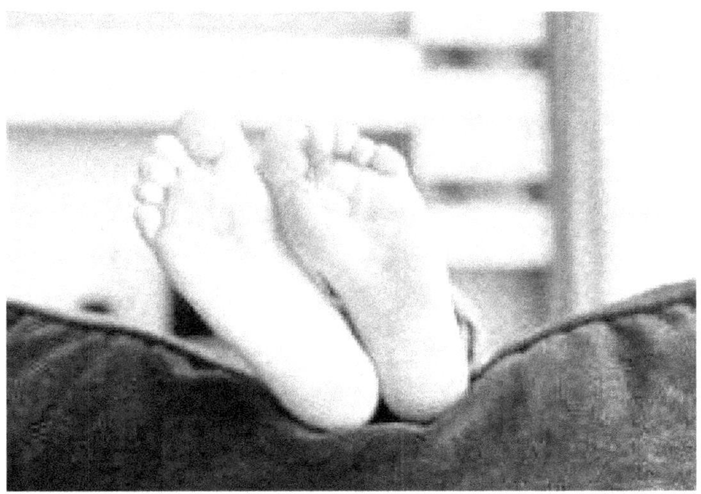

69. Where would you sleep tonight if you were

homeless?

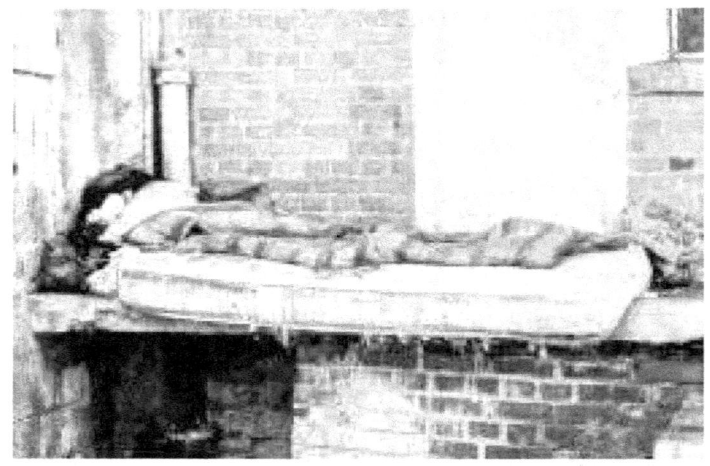

70. You are in a crowded city. Someone strapped a

ticking time bomb on your chest. You have one minute

before it explodes. Where would you go?

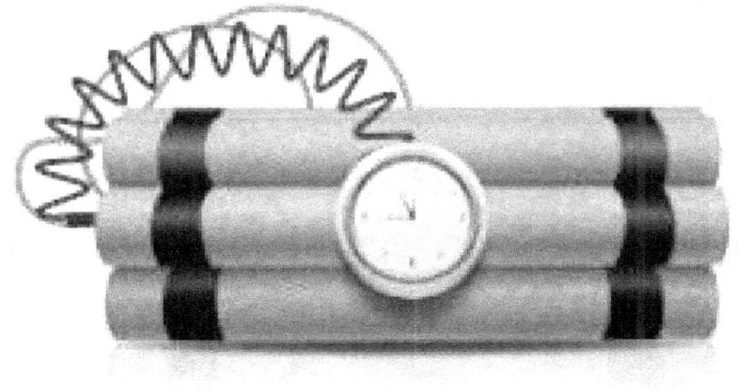

71. You are stuck in a rocket ship floating in space. You have just two minutes left to live. The whole world is watching you. What do you want to say to everyone on Earth?

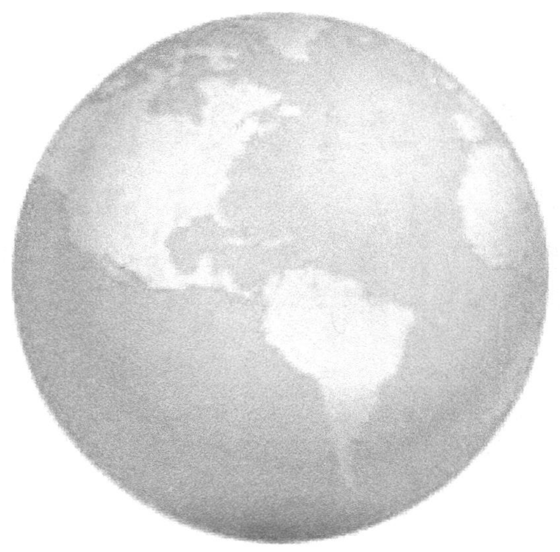

72. You have been elected President. What one law, no matter how noble or ridiculous, would you enact on your first day?

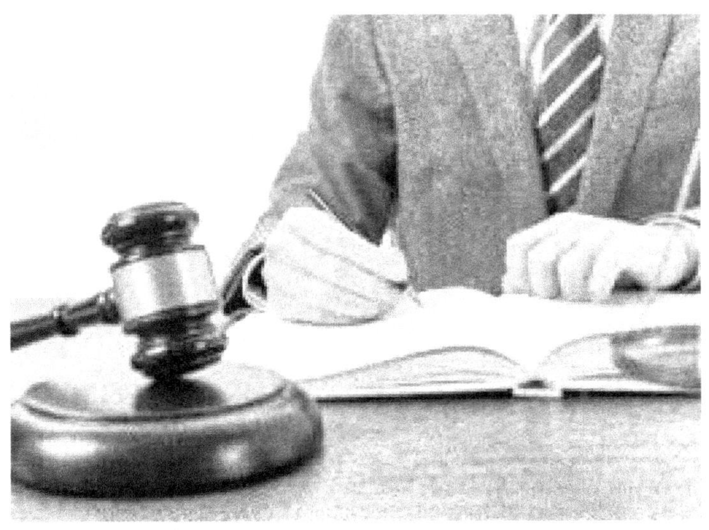

73. If you believe in God, what can convince you that there is no God?

74. If you don't believe in God, what can convince you that there is a God?

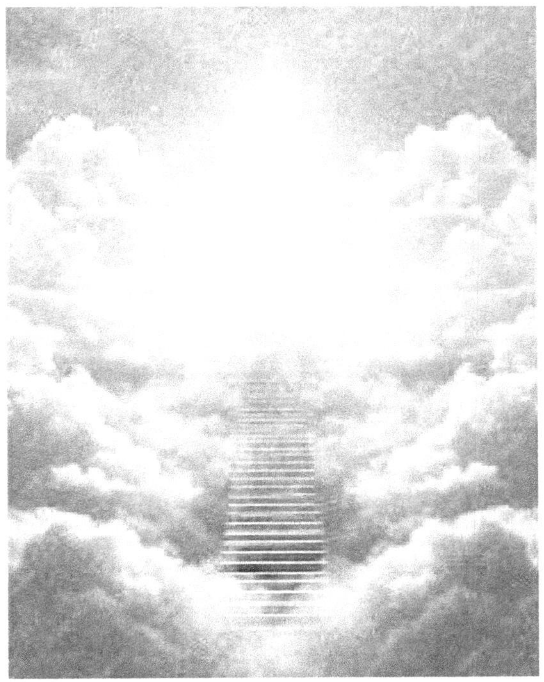

75. Say your life is a work of fiction up to this point.

The writer has ran out of ideas. How would you

complete the ending to make it interesting?

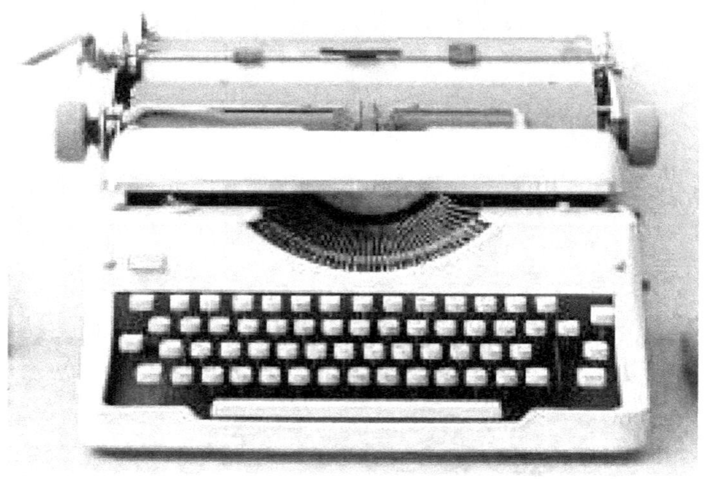

76. What one thing you wish you can stop doing right

now that will make your life ten times better?

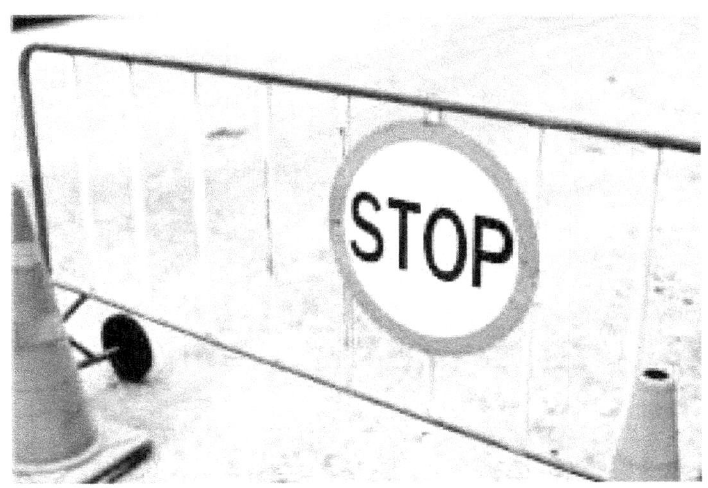

77. What if a celebrity or artist you admire has killed your entire family. Would you still admire his or her works?

78. Would you rather donate $10,000 to charity or find out later that you have overpaid for something you bought by the same amount?

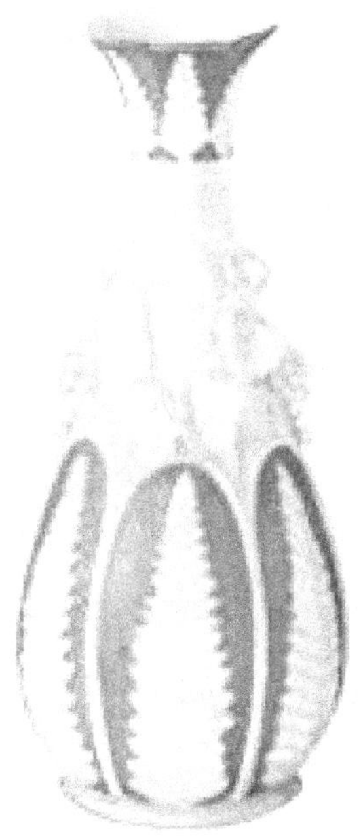

79. Over the past year, did you meet anyone new you wished you met years ago that could have changed your life then?

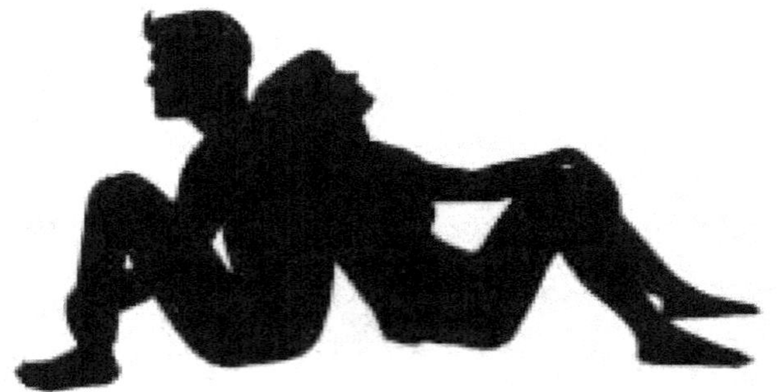

80. Do you think you are the smartest out of all the

people you know?

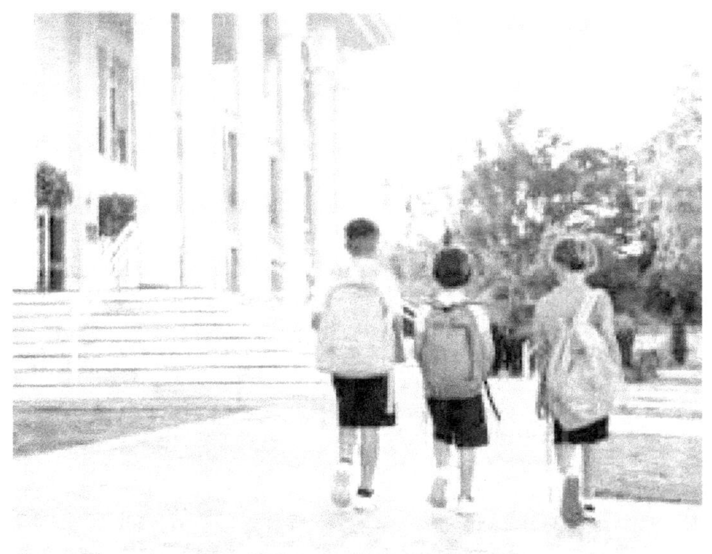

81. If you were to learn a language that no one speaks just to impress, what language would you learn?

82. Where you ever fooled by a magician into thinking

a trick was real?

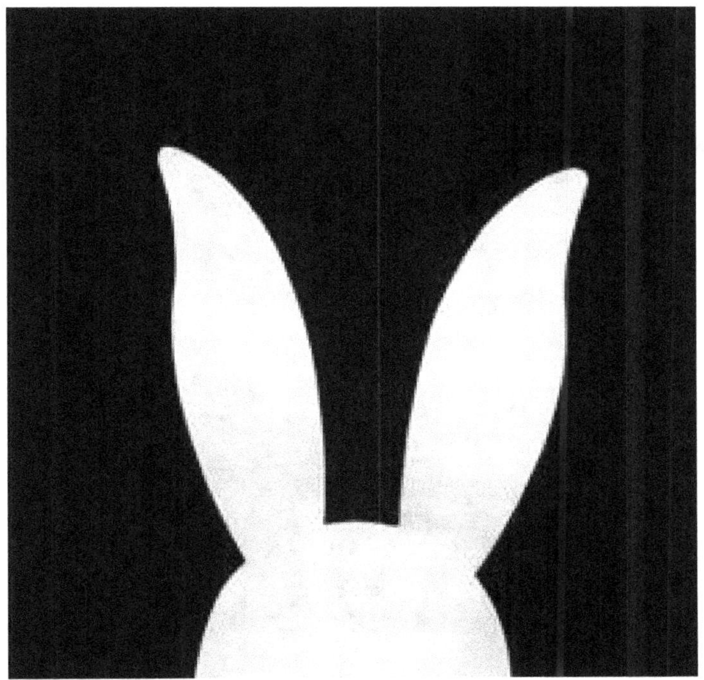

83. Have you ever went to two fortune tellers

separately to see if they both agree on your future?

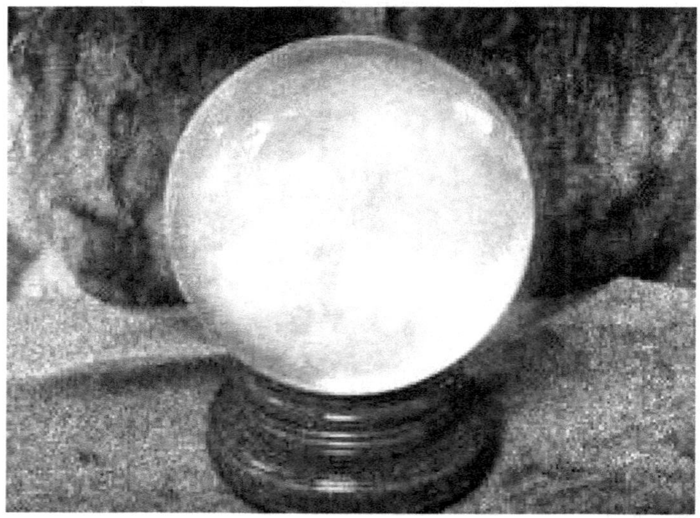

84. Why do women own so many purses?

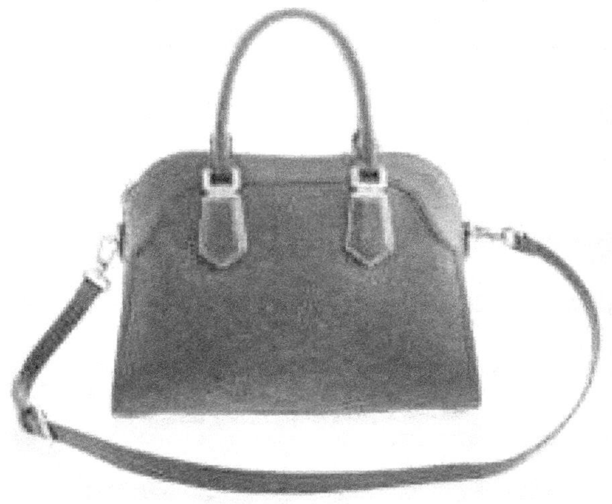

85. Have you ever tried to stay awake for 48 hours,

and did you noticed anything unusual?

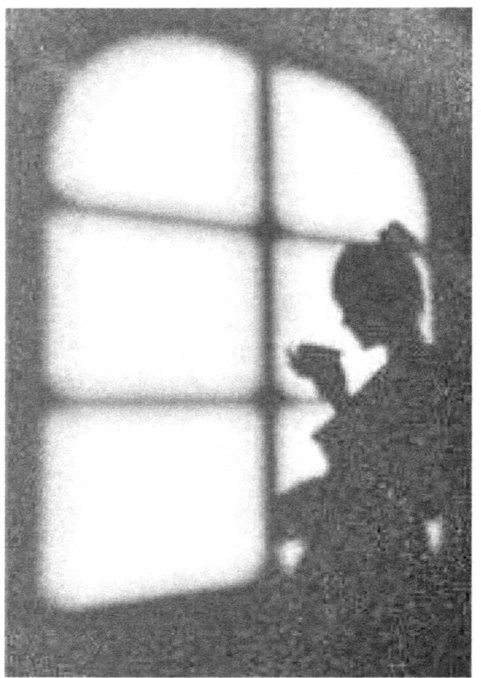

86. If you can choose a species, would you be proud to call yourself a human being or a dolphin?

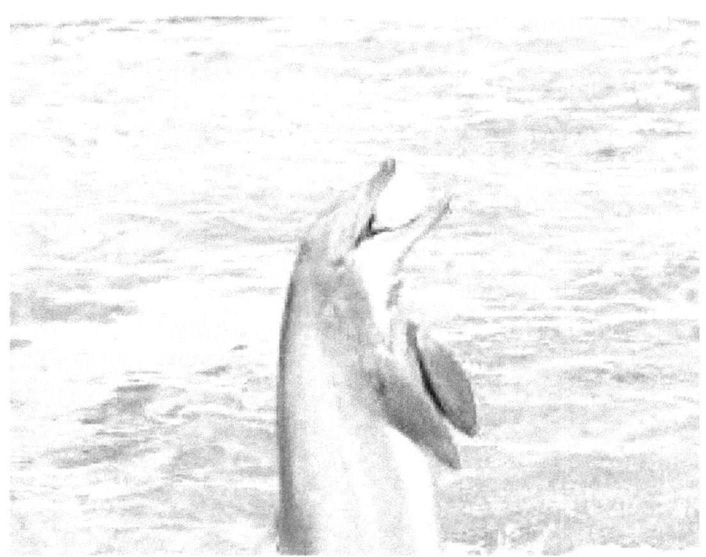

87. Have you ever followed someone around without

them knowing?

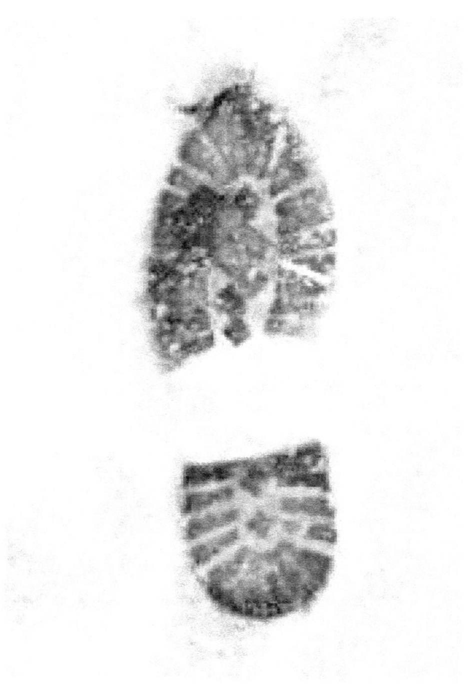

88. Do you feel any guilt from killing an insect?

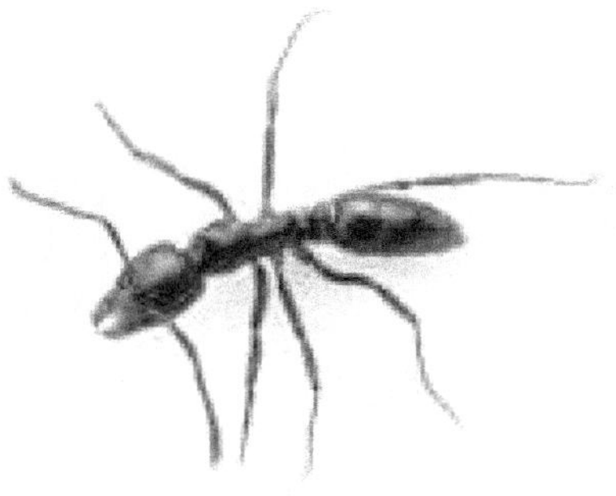

89. On your last day on Earth, how many animals do you think were killed to make all your meals in your lifetime?

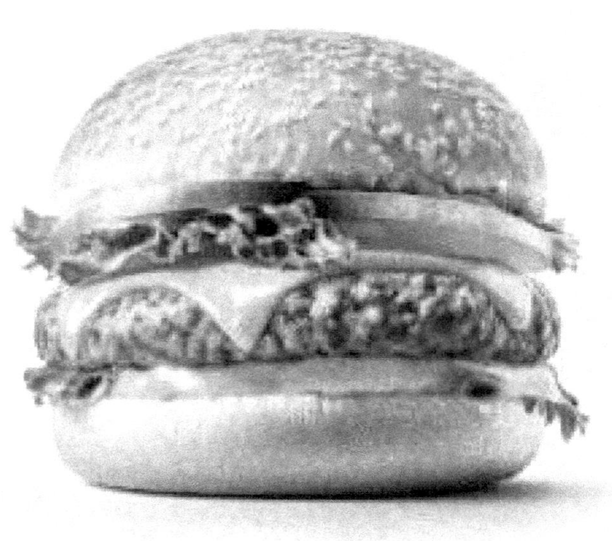

90. What album would you listen to a hundred times

straight without getting tired of it?

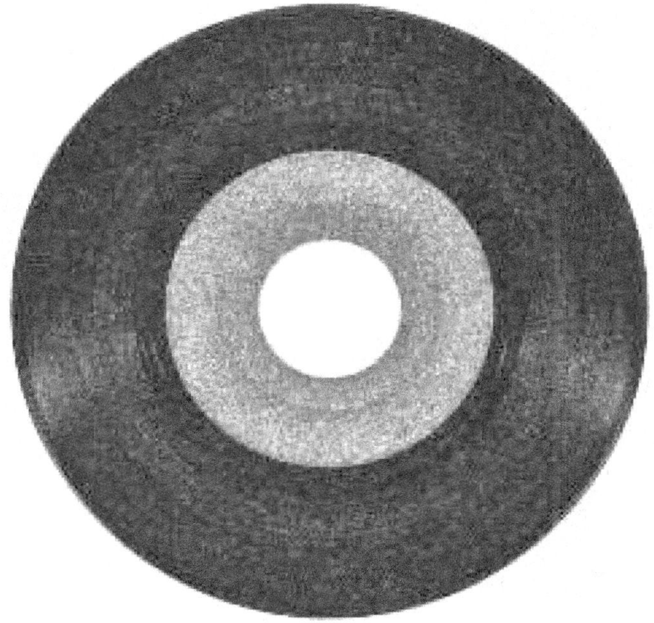

91. What was the longest time you have ever waited

for an event, and was it worth the wait?

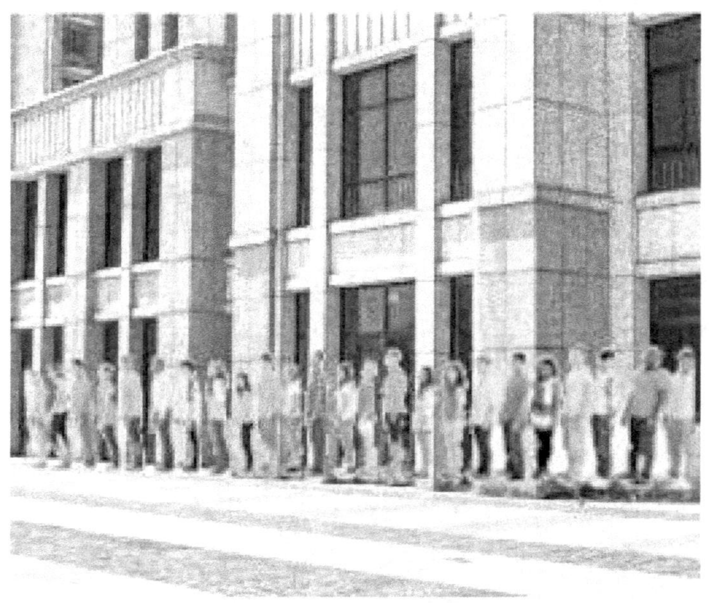

92. Would you celebrate Christmas if there were no presents involved?

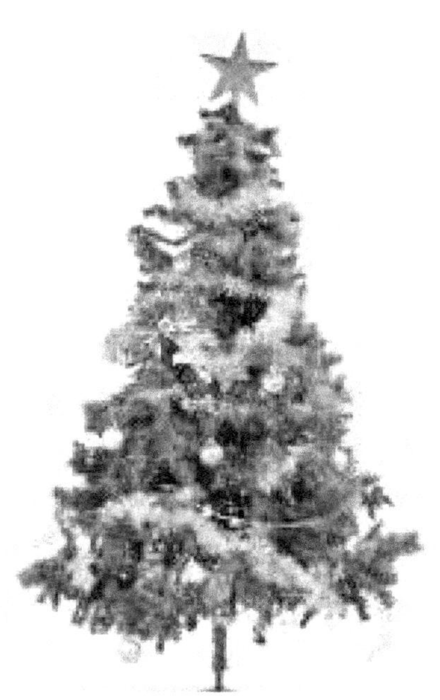

93. A UFO has crashed into your backyard, and the grass is on fire. What is the first thing you do?

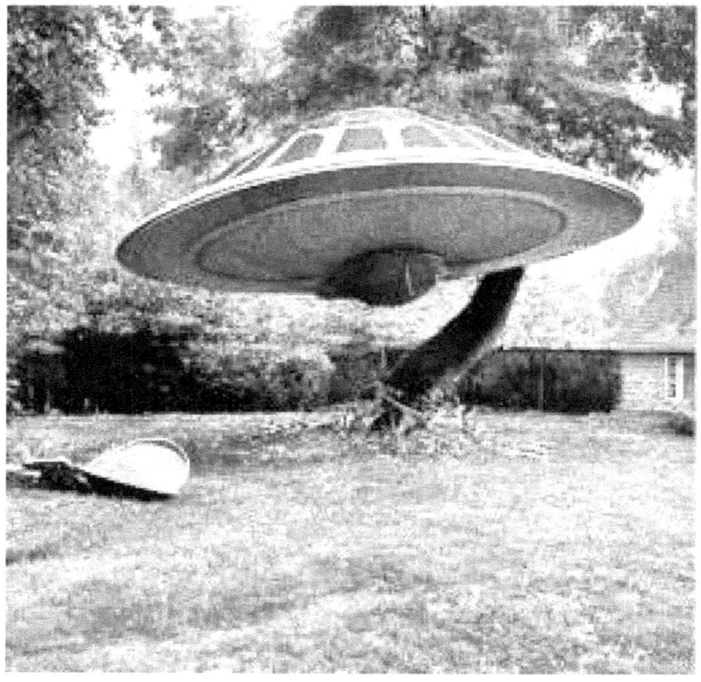

94. Your life partner decides to tell you he or she used

to be of the opposite gender. How would you react?

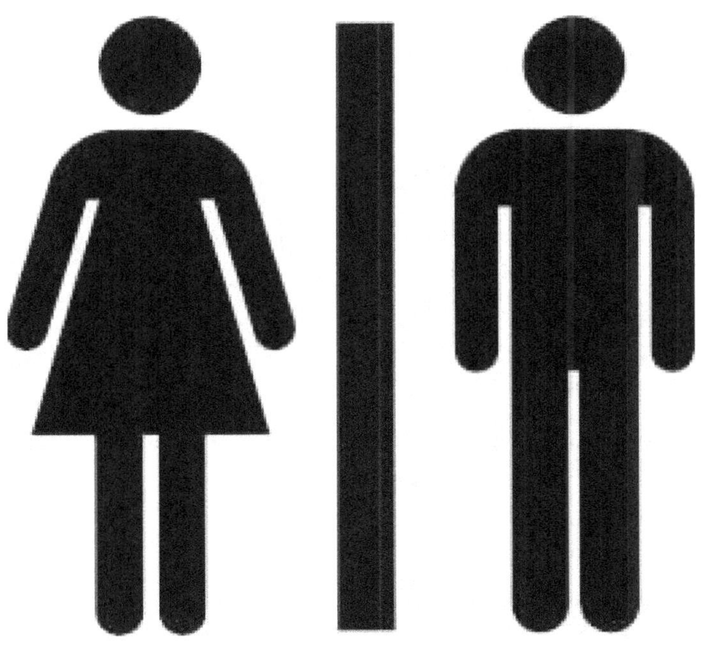

95. You happen to notice your neighbor is having an affair through the window. Your neighbor sees you looking and knows that you know. Would you confront your neighbor or your neighbor's spouse?

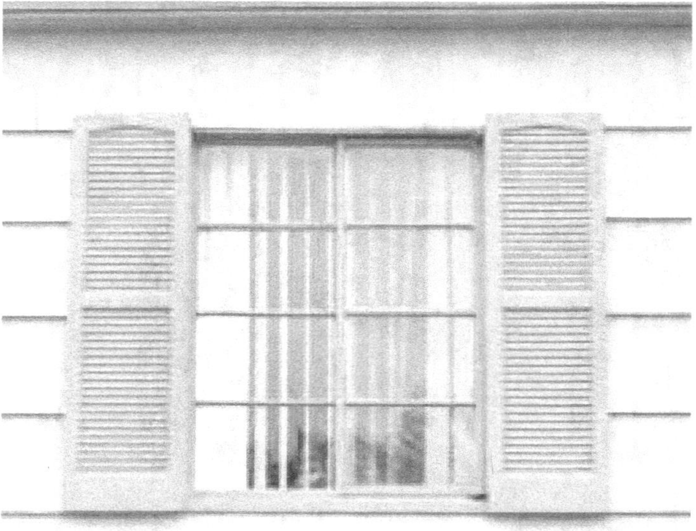

96. If you can do something 30 minutes each day to prolong your life by ten years, would you do it?

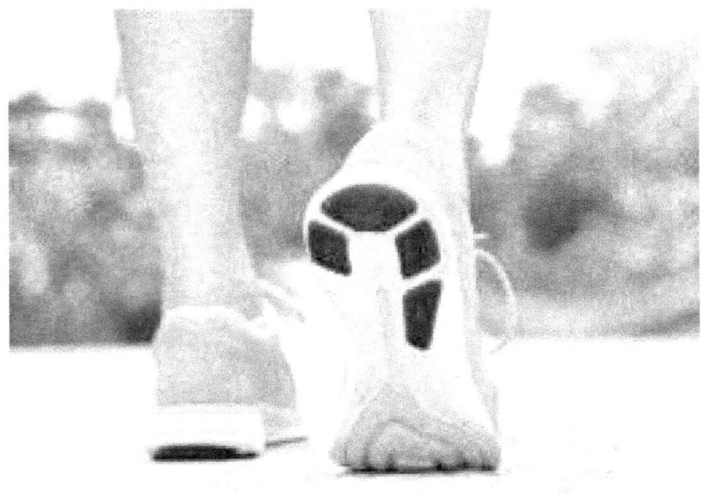

97. Would you help a homeless person even though you know what you give will be spent on alcohol?

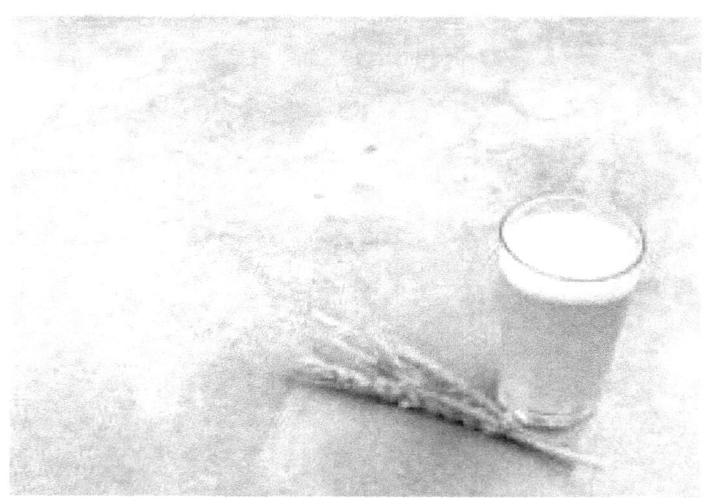

98. A loved one in your family died and left a large fortune. In order to claim it, you must renounce your religion. If you are not religious, you must convert to one. Will you do it?

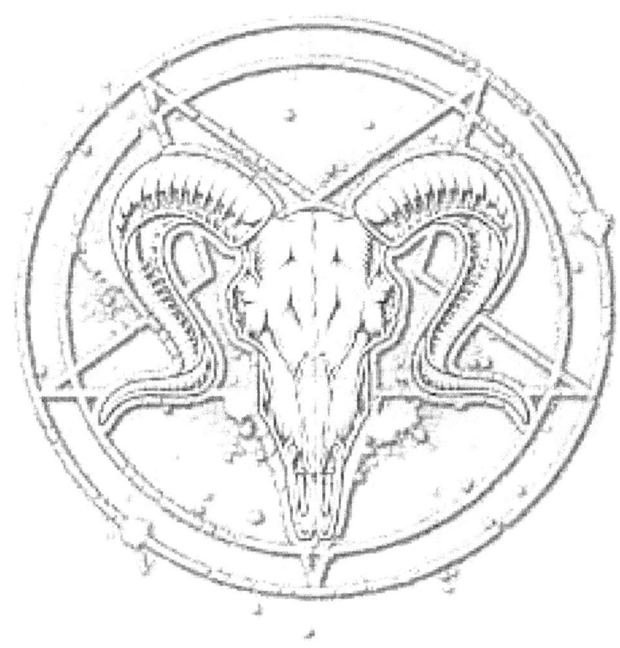

99. If you were to write a memoir, what would the
outline look like?

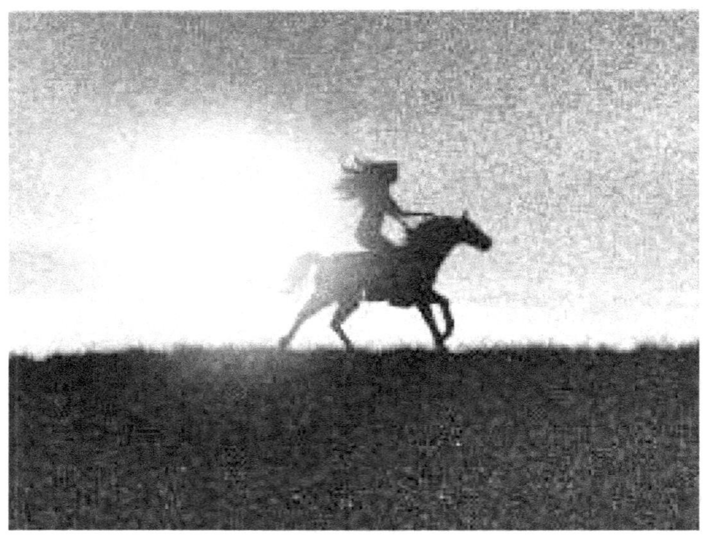

100. What one thing in the future you think is worth

staying alive for?

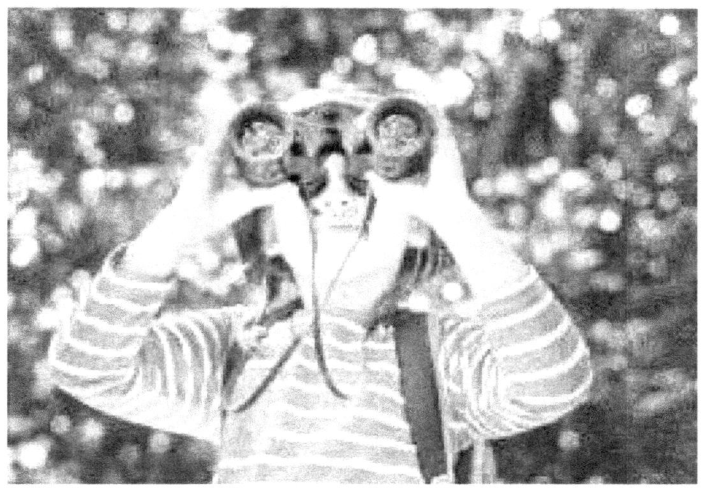

101. If the next time you fall asleep, you will never

wake up again, what will be your last thought?

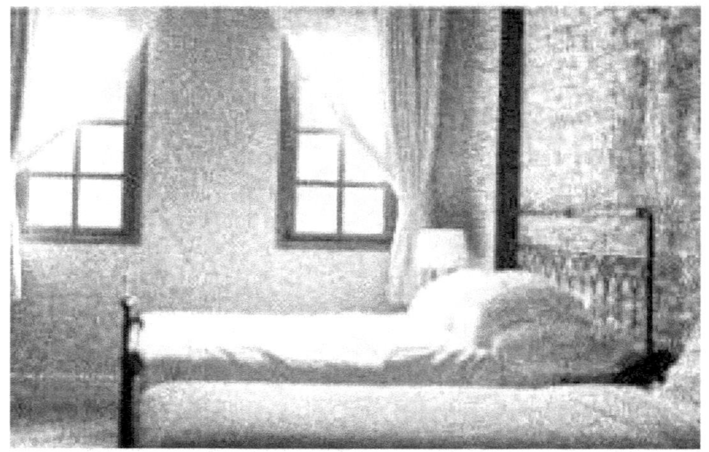

References

How was the world populated?

https://www.cea.fr/english/lists/staticfiles/clefs/science
-history/how-was-the-earth-populated.html

Can thinking intensely burn calories?

https://time.com/5400025/does-thinking-burn-calories/

Photos and artwork designed by Freepik

https://www.freepik.com/

www.ingramcontent.com/pod-product-compliance
Lightning Source LLC
Chambersburg PA
CBHW070901260726
48661CB00004B/1525